Emergency Medicine Essentials

Core Skills and Protocols for Life-Saving Care in Critical Situations

Mario F. Dennis, MD, FACEP
Attending Physician, Emergency Medicine

Copyright © 2024 by Mario F. Dennis, MD, FACEP

All rights reserved.

No part of this publication may be reproduced, distributed, or transmitted in any form or by any means, including photocopying, recording, or other electronic or mechanical methods, without the prior written permission of the publisher, except in the case of brief quotations embodied in critical reviews and certain other non-commercial uses permitted by copyright law.

Preface

The field of emergency medicine stands at the intersection of urgency, precision, and care, where moments define outcomes and decisions save lives. Emergency Medicine Essentials: Core Skills and Protocols for Life-Saving Care in Critical Situations is crafted to be an indispensable resource for healthcare providers navigating the dynamic challenges of emergency settings. It reflects the culmination of my experiences, the insights of countless colleagues, and the integration of the latest clinical guidelines and evidence-based practices.

Emergency medicine is both an art and a science. Providers must master the ability to swiftly recognize life-threatening conditions, deploy the appropriate interventions, and communicate effectively under pressure—all while maintaining compassion for patients and their families. This book is designed to serve as a practical, accessible guide to enhance these skills, bridging foundational knowledge with advanced protocols.

Purpose of the Book

This text aims to equip medical students, residents, and practicing clinicians with a structured framework for managing critical scenarios. It emphasizes the importance of a systematic approach to patient care while addressing the complexities of working in high-stakes environments. Whether dealing with anaphylaxis, cardiac arrest, severe sepsis, or intricate toxicological emergencies, the protocols and insights provided here are tailored to ensure optimal outcomes.

Key Features

General Approach: The first chapter lays the groundwork for effective emergency care by addressing essential aspects such as triage, communication with interdisciplinary teams, legal considerations, infection control, and managing special patient populations. It also highlights strategies for navigating challenging interactions, safely discharging vulnerable patients, and responding to major incidents.

Life-Threatening Emergencies: This section provides step-by-step management protocols for critical conditions such as anaphylaxis, cardiac arrest, and shock. Evidence-based algorithms and practical tips guide providers through each stage of patient stabilization and resuscitation.

Management of Critical Medical Conditions: Covering a broad spectrum of emergencies, this chapter delves into the interpretation of electrocardiograms, management of cardiovascular crises, neurological emergencies, respiratory distress, and more. Comprehensive yet concise, it ensures readers can quickly access the information needed in time-sensitive situations.

Toxicology: The final chapter addresses the principles of poison management, including diagnosis, supportive care, and the use of antidotes. Specific poisonings—ranging from opioids and acetaminophen to cyanide and carbon monoxide—are explored in detail, with practical examples to guide clinical decision-making.

Acknowledgments

This book would not have been possible without the unwavering support of my colleagues, mentors, and the patients who have trusted me with their care. I am deeply grateful to my peers in emergency medicine, whose collaborative efforts and shared experiences have profoundly shaped this work.

Conclusion

Emergency Medicine Essentials is more than a textbook; it is a tool for empowerment. It is my hope that this resource will serve as a guide in moments of uncertainty, a reference in times of crisis, and a foundation for lifelong learning. As the field of emergency medicine continues to evolve, so too must our commitment to excellence in patient care.

Mario F. Dennis, MD, FACEP
Attending Physician, Emergency Medicine

Preface
Table of contents
List of Abbreviations

Table of Contents

Chapter 1: General Approach

1. Scope of the Emergency Department
    - Note-Keeping
    - Radiological Requests
    - Triage
    - Discharge, Referral, and Handover

2. Interprofessional Collaboration
    - Working with General Practitioners (GPs)
    - Providing Telephone Advice
    - Coordination with Ambulance Crews

3. Managing Unique Challenges
    - Navigating as a Junior Doctor
    - Handling Inappropriate Attendances

- Supporting Patients with Preexisting Labels or Special Needs
- Discharging Elderly Patients Safely
- Communicating Bad News and Death Protocols

4. Legal and Infection Control Considerations
   - Legal Risks and Law Overview
   - Infection Control and Prevention

5. Emergency Responses Outside the ED
   - Essential Supplies for On-the-Go Care
   - Roadside Emergencies and Major Incident Responses

Chapter 2: Life-Threatening Emergencies

1. Anaphylaxis
   - Overview and Treatment Algorithm

2. Choking
   - Airway Obstruction Management

3. Cardiac Arrest

- Recognition and Management
- Resuscitation Algorithms (Basic and Advanced)
- Post-Resuscitation Care

4. Critical Procedures
   - Central Venous Access
   - Advanced Life Support Algorithm

5. Sepsis and Shock
   - Recognition and Early Management

Chapter 3: Management of Critical Medical Conditions

1. Cardiovascular and Respiratory Emergencies
   - ECG Interpretation for ACS and Arrhythmias
   - Management of Hypertensive Emergencies, Pulmonary Edema, and Dyspnea

2. Neurological and Endocrine Crises

- Stroke, Seizures, Delirium, Thyrotoxic and Addisonian Crisis

3. Gastrointestinal and Renal Emergencies
   - GI Bleeds, Acute Renal Failure, Electrolyte Disturbances

4. Hematological Emergencies
   - Coagulopathies, Sickle Cell Disease, Transfusion Protocols

Chapter 4: Toxicology

1. General Principles
   - Diagnosing and Managing Poisoned Patients
   - Supportive Care and Reducing Poison Absorption

2. Antidotes
   - Mechanisms, Indications, and Case Applications

3. Specific Poisonings

- Opioids, Salicylates, Paracetamol, TCAs, Benzodiazepines, Barbiturates
- Lithium, Beta-Blockers, Digoxin, and More

4. Special Cases
    - Cyanide, Organophosphates, Carbon Monoxide, and Chlorine Poisonings

List of Abbreviations

ACLS – Advanced Cardiovascular Life Support

AED – Automated External Defibrillator

ALS – Advanced Life Support

ATLS – Advanced Trauma Life Support

BLS – Basic Life Support

BP – Blood Pressure

BVM – Bag-Valve-Mask

CAB – Circulation, Airway, Breathing

CPR – Cardiopulmonary Resuscitation

CXR – Chest X-Ray

DNR – Do Not Resuscitate

DOA – Dead on Arrival

ED – Emergency Department

ECG/EKG – Electrocardiogram

ETT – Endotracheal Tube

FAST – Focused Assessment with Sonography for Trauma

GCS – Glasgow Coma Scale

HR – Heart Rate

HTN – Hypertension

IV – Intravenous

IO – Intraosseous

LOC – Level of Consciousness

MI – Myocardial Infarction

MVC – Motor Vehicle Collision

O2 – Oxygen

PE – Pulmonary Embolism

PPE – Personal Protective Equipment

PR – Pulse Rate

ROSC – Return of Spontaneous Circulation

RR – Respiratory Rate

SIRS – Systemic Inflammatory Response Syndrome

STEMI – ST-Elevation Myocardial Infarction

SVT – Supraventricular Tachycardia

TIA – Transient Ischemic Attack

TBI – Traumatic Brain Injury

TTE – Transthoracic Echocardiogram

VF – Ventricular Fibrillation

VT – Ventricular Tachycardia

WBC – White Blood Cell

Chapter 1

General Approach

This outline organizes key topics relevant to emergency department practice, emphasizing practical aspects of patient care, communication, legal considerations, and crisis response. Each section aims to provide guidance for healthcare professionals navigating complex, high-pressure environments.

Scope of the Emergency Department

1. Note-Keeping
2. Radiological Requests
3. Triage
4. Discharge, Referral, and Handover
5. Collaborating with General Practitioners (GPs)
6. Providing Telephone Advice
7. Coordination with Ambulance Crews
8. Navigating as a Junior Doctor

9. Addressing Inappropriate Attendances
10. Managing Patients with Preexisting Labels
11. Handling Challenging Patient Interactions
12. Caring for Special Patient Populations
13. Safely Discharging Elderly Patients
14. Supporting Patients with Learning Disabilities
15. Facilitating Patient Transfers
16. Communicating Bad News
17. Procedures Following a Death
18. Legal Considerations: Minimizing Risks
19. Legal Considerations: Understanding the Law
20. Infection Control and Prevention Measures
21. Essential Supplies for On-the-Go Medical Situations
22. Managing Roadside Emergencies
23. Responding to Major Incidents

The Role and Function of the Emergency Department (ED)

The Emergency Department (ED) serves as a critical intersection between primary and secondary care. It functions as a highly visible component of the healthcare system, often accessed directly by patients without prior referral. Referrals may also originate from various sources, including general practitioners (GPs), NHS Direct, minor injury units, and other healthcare providers. The ED addresses a wide range of medical conditions, focusing primarily on acute and distressing illnesses or injuries.

Primary Responsibilities of the ED

The ED's primary responsibilities include:

1. Delivering life-saving interventions promptly.

2. Alleviating pain through appropriate analgesia.

3. Initiating necessary investigations and treatments.

4. Determining the need for admission or discharge.

Interdisciplinary Collaboration

ED operations rely on a multidisciplinary team approach, emphasizing clinical competency over traditional roles. Key personnel include:

Nurses: Nurse practitioners, consultants, and healthcare assistants.

Doctors: Permanent and temporary staff.

Administrative Team: Receptionists, managers, and secretaries.

Specialist Staff: Radiographers, psychiatric liaison nurses, plaster technicians, physiotherapists, paramedic practitioners, and occupational therapists.

Support Personnel: Security staff, porters, and cleaners.

Infrastructure and Resources

The ED is designed to handle a spectrum of emergencies, with facilities that cater to diverse needs. Core areas include:

Resuscitation Rooms: For critically ill or injured patients.

Observation Areas: For patients on trolleys requiring monitoring.

Ambulatory Sections: For minor injuries and non-critical conditions.

Specialized Zones: Separate areas for pediatric care, wound management, imaging, and eye examinations.

Patient Flow and Discharge Options

Efficient patient flow is crucial for ED functionality. Discharge pathways include:

1. Home without follow-up: For minor issues.

2. Home with follow-up: Involving GPs or community services.

3. Hospital clinic follow-up: Arranged for ongoing care.

4. Hospital admission: For further treatment.

5. Specialized transfer: To facilities with advanced care capabilities.

Extended Roles of ED Staff

Beyond direct patient care, ED professionals contribute to various healthcare settings:

Short-Stay Wards: For observation and early discharge planning.

Outpatient Clinics: Managing conditions like burns, infections, or fractures.

Operating Theaters: Handling specific surgical cases, such as simple fractures.

Telemedicine: Providing remote guidance to satellite units.

Emergency Care Across Settings

As emergency care evolves, patients now receive treatment in diverse settings, including minor injury units, acute medical assessment units, and walk-in centers. This development has blurred the lines between emergency medicine, acute care, and primary healthcare.

Documentation in the ED: A Critical Component

Accurate, thorough, and legible documentation is indispensable for patient care and legal purposes. The ED record is often the primary evidence in negligence cases. Adherence to professional standards in note-keeping reflects the quality of care provided.

Key Guidelines for Note-Keeping

1. Record all relevant history, examination findings, and clinical decisions.

2. Ensure legibility and clarity, avoiding abbreviations and judgmental terms.

3. Document medications, including dosage, timing, and administration route.

4. Outline discharge instructions, follow-up arrangements, and red flags.

5. Always include the date, time, and signature with printed name and designation.

Radiological Requests and Reporting

Radiological imaging is a critical diagnostic tool in the ED, but requests should align with clinical guidelines to avoid unnecessary exposure or litigation concerns. Radiological findings are reviewed promptly, and abnormalities are flagged for immediate attention.

Radiological Request Best Practices

Provide clear clinical indications and suspected diagnoses.

Avoid unnecessary imaging, relying instead on clinical evaluation and established guidelines.

Consider pregnancy risks in relevant cases and consult senior staff when needed.

Triage in Emergency Departments: Evidence-Based Perspectives

Triage is an essential process in emergency departments (EDs) designed to prioritize patients based on the severity of their condition and the availability of departmental resources. This ensures that those with life-threatening conditions receive care first. One widely implemented approach is the National Triage Scale, which categorizes patients into different levels of urgency.

Triage Process: Key Aspects

1. Initial Assessment by Triage Nurse:
Upon arrival, patients are quickly evaluated by a senior, experienced triage nurse. This brief assessment typically includes basic interventions (e.g., splinting injuries, applying ice packs, or administering pain relief) and initiating necessary investigations such as ordering X-rays to expedite care.

2. Dynamic Nature of Triage:
The urgency assigned to a patient can evolve over time. For instance, a middle-aged patient presenting with an ankle sprain may initially be categorized as low urgency (green). However, if the patient later exhibits symptoms like chest

pain or sweating, they would require reclassification to a higher priority (orange) for immediate care.

3. Misconceptions About Triage Categories:
Triage assignments do not equate to a diagnosis or indicate the long-term prognosis. For example, an elderly patient with severe abdominal discomfort may be placed in a moderate urgency category (yellow) due to current stability, even though the underlying condition (e.g., metastatic cancer causing bowel obstruction) may carry a grave prognosis.

4. Challenges in Triage:
Non-urgent cases often experience longer waiting times, potentially causing dissatisfaction. Elderly or uncomplaining patients may be inadvertently overlooked. It is crucial to manage expectations by informing patients about likely delays and ensuring their comfort and safety during the wait.

Discharge, Referral, and Continuity of Care

1. Discharge Process:
Most patients treated in the ED are discharged home with instructions for follow-up care, often involving a general practitioner (GP). Patients should be provided with clear verbal and written instructions on when and why to seek further medical help. This is particularly important for individuals with minor head injuries or immobilized limbs, where monitoring for complications is crucial.

2. Patient Referrals to Inpatient Teams:
Referral decisions depend on the severity of the case. For example, a patient with a suspected myocardial infarction would require urgent admission, whereas borderline cases (e.g., atypical chest pain with normal investigations) may necessitate further assessment. Before referring, ED staff should ensure:

Appropriate investigations (e.g., ECGs, X-rays) have been conducted.

Necessary treatments, such as pain relief, have been provided without delay.

A concise summary of the patient's history, investigations, and treatment is ready for the inpatient team.

3. Communication During Referrals:
When referring a patient, clarity is vital:

Identify yourself and the specialist's name and grade.

Clearly state whether the referral is for admission or consultation.

In case of disagreement over admission, escalate concerns to senior ED staff for resolution.

4. Documentation:
Comprehensive and legible notes ensure continuity of care, especially when pending test results need follow-up. Specialists attending the

patient should also document their findings and plans in the ED notes.

Handover Between Healthcare Providers

1. Challenges of Patient Handover:
Handover at the end of a shift can lead to oversight if not managed carefully. Ideally, ED staff should complete care plans or referrals before leaving. If delays occur (e.g., pending test results), ensure a thorough handover to the incoming team.

2. Effective Handover Practices:
Include all pertinent details, such as the patient's history, investigation results, and treatment provided. Inform the patient that their care will be continued by another clinician to maintain trust.

Role of General Practitioners (GPs) in ED Care

GPs play a pivotal role in coordinating patient care, especially for individuals with complex social or medical needs. They can provide essential insights into a patient's history and home circumstances, guiding decisions on admission or discharge. For example:

A frail elderly patient with a wrist fracture may require home support or hospital admission, depending on their home situation and support network.

When a GP refers a patient for admission, the ED team should consult them before discharge to ensure alignment with the patient's overall care plan.

Telephone Consultations and Telemedicine in Emergency Care

1. Telephone Advice:
Calls from patients or caregivers should be handled with the same diligence as face-to-face consultations. Record all details, including the patient's condition, advice given, and caller's

information, ensuring comprehensive documentation.

2. Telemedicine:

Telemedicine facilitates access to emergency care in rural or remote areas. Through video consultations and teleradiology, senior ED staff can provide specialist advice or determine the need for interventions such as fracture manipulations. Accurate documentation and adherence to protocols are essential for safe telemedicine practices.

In conclusion, effective triage, discharge planning, and communication with other healthcare providers are critical components of ED care. These processes ensure timely treatment, patient safety, and seamless transitions between different levels of care.

Coping as a Junior Doctor in the Emergency Department

Physical Demands of the Job

Transitioning into the Emergency Department (ED) as a junior doctor, even with over a year of experience, can be a daunting challenge. The reality, however, often proves less intimidating than anticipated. While the total hours worked may seem fewer than in other specialties, the intensity of the workload makes ED roles physically and mentally demanding. Shifts typically involve prolonged periods of standing, walking, decision-making, and constant alertness, leaving doctors physically drained by the end of their duty. Maintaining a healthy balance between professional responsibilities and personal life is crucial, as overextending in both areas is unsustainable. Rest and relaxation during off-duty hours are essential to replenish energy and maintain optimal performance. Fatigue impairs judgment, increases the likelihood of errors, and fosters interpersonal conflicts, emphasizing the importance of self-care.

Mental Challenges and Decision-Making

The mental demands of emergency medicine are considerable, particularly for those unaccustomed to making independent, definitive decisions based on their own assessments and investigations. While initially overwhelming, decision-making becomes more manageable with practice and a structured approach. After taking a history and conducting a physical examination, junior doctors should systematically address key questions:

What is the likely diagnosis?

What investigations are necessary to confirm it?

What treatments are required, and do I have the necessary skills?

Does the patient require referral or specialist review?

Recognizing one's limitations is as important as making confident decisions. Seeking timely assistance from senior staff or specialists is a vital skill, especially in complex cases. When facing uncooperative specialists or inadequate advice, advocate firmly for the patient's best interests, involving senior ED staff as needed.

Continuous Learning and Professional Growth

Every shift presents opportunities for learning. Junior doctors should actively engage with cases, documenting interesting or complex conditions for post-shift review. Seeking guidance from senior colleagues and utilizing department resources fosters professional development. Dedicating time to reading about new conditions encountered enhances both confidence and competence.

Building Strong Team Relationships

Emergency medicine thrives on teamwork. Respect for colleagues, regardless of their role or tenure, is fundamental. Demonstrating humility and a willingness to contribute, even in tasks outside one's formal responsibilities, fosters camaraderie and mutual respect. For instance, assisting with patient transport during busy periods not only supports the team but also benefits patient care.

Managing Shifts and Maintaining Well-Being

Punctuality and reliability are non-negotiable in the ED. Inform senior staff promptly if unable to work, and ensure regular breaks during shifts to maintain energy levels. Proper hydration, nutrition, and rest are critical for sustained performance. Interpersonal challenges with colleagues should be set aside during work hours, prioritizing professionalism and patient care.

Coping with Stress and Seeking Support

Feelings of being overwhelmed are not uncommon, and acknowledging this is crucial. Open communication with senior staff, consultants, or support services can provide valuable relief and guidance. Ignoring these emotions risks personal well-being and compromises patient safety. Confidential resources, such as counseling services, are available for doctors needing additional support.

Managing Common ED Challenges

Addressing Inappropriate Attendances

Patients presenting to the ED with conditions better suited for primary care remain a contentious issue. Such cases may constitute 4–20% of ED visits, influenced by factors like patient perceptions, access to primary care, and regional healthcare practices. While it is vital to address these cases appropriately, labeling them as "inappropriate" can be counterproductive. Educating patients and implementing systems like minor injury units or embedded GP services can help manage this workload effectively.

Handling Referrals and Patient Labels

Referrals from other practitioners or patients self-identifying with specific conditions require careful evaluation. While referral letters are valuable, they should not be accepted uncritically, as clinical presentations may evolve. Self-labeled patients often possess deep knowledge about their conditions, and respecting their input fosters trust and improves outcomes. Similarly, frequent ED visitors require thorough assessment each time to avoid missing critical diagnoses. For complex cases, collaborative planning involving social services, primary care, and psychiatric teams may be necessary.

Navigating Difficult Patient Interactions

Junior doctors will inevitably encounter challenging patients. Factors such as medical conditions, social circumstances, or substance use often contribute to difficult interactions. Maintaining professionalism, empathy, and an open mind is essential. Recognize that these situations are not personal and remain focused on providing quality care.

Discharging Elderly Patients

Identifying individuals at risk after hospital discharge requires evaluating both medical and social factors rather than following strict predisposing criteria. Factors influencing post-discharge challenges include the primary medical condition, existing comorbidities, functional status, and social circumstances.

Indicators of Risk

Elderly patients often have multiple comorbidities and atypical symptoms, making them more susceptible to the consequences of acute illness. Key risk indicators include:

Medical History and Current Condition: Patients with dementia, psychiatric illnesses, or significant changes in physical or mental health require careful consideration. Recent events, such as bereavement or a decline in cognitive ability, may signal additional vulnerabilities.

Living Situation: Those living alone or lacking family support are at higher risk, especially if their home environment is unsuitable (e.g., stairs, mobility challenges).

Self-Neglect: Signs of poor hygiene, inappropriate clothing, weight loss, or unexplained bruising may indicate difficulties managing at home or more severe underlying issues like malignancy or frequent falls.

Assessment of Coping Ability

Evaluating an elderly person's ability to manage independently involves identifying self-neglect, mobility issues, and behavioral changes. Input from relatives, general practitioners (GPs), or community care providers is crucial. For instance, unexplained weight loss might indicate challenges with meal preparation or access to food, while frequent falls could necessitate a falls clinic assessment to address contributing factors like poor lighting or unsuitable footwear.

Discharge Planning

Hospitalization can disorient elderly patients, making discharge to their familiar home environment preferable, provided concerns about their functional and cognitive abilities are addressed. Occupational and physiotherapy assessments, along with home evaluations, can identify necessary adaptations and equipment. Involving community services (e.g., district nurses, social workers, rapid response teams) is essential to prevent future complications.

Caring for Patients with Learning Difficulties

Patients with learning disabilities often present complex health needs, with higher healthcare utilization rates than the general population. Their care requires specialized communication techniques and a thorough understanding of their medical and behavioral needs.

Common Associated Health Issues

Patients with learning difficulties are predisposed to specific health problems, including:

Sensory impairments (vision, hearing).

Gastrointestinal conditions (e.g., reflux, constipation).

Increased risk of infections and epilepsy.

Mental health disorders (e.g., depression, schizophrenia), with syndromic associations such as dementia in Down syndrome.

Leading Causes of Mortality

Conditions like pneumonia, linked to swallowing difficulties and aspiration, and congenital heart disease are prevalent causes of death in this population. Recognizing these risks early can guide preventive and therapeutic strategies.

Effective Communication

Successful consultations require adapting to the patient's communication abilities:

Start by explaining the consultation process and engaging the patient directly before involving caregivers.

Use simplified language and questions tied to familiar events (e.g., "Did this start before lunch?").

Behavioral changes often indicate health issues since patients may struggle to articulate symptoms.

Patient Transfers

Transferring patients between facilities requires meticulous planning to ensure safety and continuity of care.

Preparation for Transfer

Before transfer, stabilize life-threatening conditions and complete a secondary assessment. Procedures like securing the airway, placing chest drains, and considering urinary catheterization should be performed as necessary.

Communication and Coordination

Clear communication with the receiving facility is critical. Provide detailed patient information, including:

Medical history and treatments administered.

Results of key investigations.

Contact information for referring and receiving clinicians.

Transport and Monitoring

During transit, ensure adequate monitoring, including ECG, pulse oximetry, and blood pressure measurement. For intubated patients, monitor end-tidal CO_2 levels. Carry sufficient emergency supplies, including oxygen, and secure all equipment and the patient safely.

Documentation

Essential documents accompanying the patient include:

Medical history, examination findings, and test results.

Details of fluids, medications, and procedures.

Contact details of involved medical personnel.

Breaking Bad News

Communicating life-threatening or fatal outcomes in emergency settings requires empathy, professionalism, and a structured approach.

Preparation

Designate a private, comfortable space for relatives, equipped with basic amenities. A dedicated staff member should accompany and support relatives, offering updates about the patient's condition and documenting key details.

Delivering the News

The task should be undertaken by experienced personnel with communication skills and authority. Steps include:

Preparing oneself (e.g., appearance, reviewing patient details).

Introducing oneself and addressing relatives by name.

Clearly and compassionately explaining the patient's condition or outcome.

Follow-Up Support

After conveying the news, remain available for questions and provide practical support, such as coordinating transportation for relatives or arranging spiritual care if needed.

Intra-Hospital Transfers

The principles of intra-hospital transfers mirror inter-hospital transfers but involve shorter distances. The focus remains on patient safety, proper communication, and timely execution to prevent delays in care.

What to Do After a Death

Key Actions Post-Death

1. Notify Authorities for Suspicious Deaths

Report suspicious deaths immediately to the police, who will coordinate with the Coroner or Procurator Fiscal (in Scotland).

2. Essential Contacts After Death in the Emergency Department (ED)

Inform the Next of Kin (NOK): If the NOK is not present, the police may assist in notifying them.

Notify the Coroner or Procurator Fiscal (in Scotland): Ensure timely reporting.

Contact the Patient's General Practitioner (GP): Inform them of the death.

Cancel Scheduled Medical Appointments: Prevent unnecessary communication.

Update Social and Health Teams: Notify social workers or health visitors if relevant.

3. Supporting the Family

Provide clear information about death certification, registration, and funeral planning.

Share educational leaflets if available.

Offer counseling resources or refer them to the GP for continued bereavement support.

Provide the ED's contact details for follow-up questions or assistance.

Information Required for Reporting to the Coroner/Procurator Fiscal

Full patient details: name, address, and date of birth.

Contact information for the next of kin.

GP details.

ED arrival and death times.

Certifying doctor's name and role.

Incident specifics, including injuries or illnesses.

Relevant medical history.

Last doctor visit details: If the patient was recently seen for a terminal condition (e.g., cancer), the GP or hospital doctor may issue a death certificate.

Religious considerations: Some faiths require expedited burials, but sudden deaths may delay this process.

Communication challenges: Highlight issues like language barriers or hearing impairments.

Addressing Staff Well-Being

Acknowledge the emotional impact of patient deaths, particularly during stressful situations or those with personal resonance.

Allow staff brief breaks after challenging scenarios, such as informing parents of a child's death.

Encourage peer and professional support for staff distressed by critical events or resuscitation failures.

Organ Donation Considerations

Identify potential organ donors, particularly in cases of unexpected cardiac arrest or patients with non-survivable conditions.

Collaborate with transplant teams and Coroners to arrange donations where feasible.

Engage specialist organ donation nurses for guidance and support.

Refer to the British Transplantation Society for more details on organ donation protocols.

Responsibilities

1. Maintaining Professionalism

Approach patients and families with empathy and transparency.

Address delays or errors honestly.

2. Consent Management

Use consent forms for complex or high-risk procedures.

Prioritize life-saving treatments while seeking consent when possible.

3. Comprehensive Documentation

Maintain clear, accurate, and contemporaneous notes.

Document injuries, investigations, referrals, and patient advice.

Label all associated documents (e.g., test results, ECGs).

4. Managing Referrals and Returns

Record referral details, including time and doctor consulted.

Treat returning patients as new cases to avoid reliance on prior diagnoses.

5. Handling Discharge Against Advice

Encourage patients to follow medical recommendations.

Document refusals thoroughly and ensure patients deemed incompetent are safeguarded.

Additional Considerations

1. Mental Capacity Act (2005)

A patient lacks capacity if unable to understand, retain, or process information or communicate decisions due to cognitive impairments.

2. Patient Records Access

Patients in the UK have a legal right to access their medical records under the Data Protection Act (1998).

3. Police Requests and Legal Compliance

Disclose information to police only with patient consent or in specific legal circumstances (e.g., Road Traffic Act violations, terrorism suspicions).

Ensure police statements are factual, concise, and devoid of opinion or conjecture.

4. Medical Defense Coverage

Membership in organizations like MDU or MPS offers essential support for legal and professional challenges, including inquiries, negligence claims, and GMC investigations.

Infection Control and Prevention

Effective infection control is critical in the Emergency Department (ED) to safeguard patients, relatives, and healthcare providers. The ED serves as a high-risk environment for the transmission of various infectious agents, including Staphylococcus aureus (e.g., MRSA), which can spread through contaminated hands or equipment, potentially infecting wounds, fractures, or in-dwelling devices like catheters or chest drains. Bloodborne pathogens such as hepatitis B, hepatitis C, and HIV pose additional risks, particularly during exposure to infected blood. Viral gastroenteritis, typically spread via the fecal-oral route, can also contaminate surfaces through vomiting, increasing transmission risk to staff and other patients.

Respiratory infections, including influenza, respiratory syncytial virus (RSV), and severe acute respiratory syndrome (SARS), spread via respiratory droplets from coughing or sneezing. Nebulizers used on infected individuals can further aerosolized these pathogens, as seen during the SARS outbreak in Hong Kong in 2003, which significantly impacted ED personnel.

Standard Precautions for Infection Prevention

Universal precautions, also known as standard precautions, are vital to minimizing infection risks in healthcare settings. These measures assume all blood and body fluids to be potentially infectious. Key components include:

1. Hand Hygiene:

Essential before and after patient contact or any activity that may contaminate hands.

Hands visibly dirty or heavily contaminated must be washed with soap and water, followed by thorough drying.

Alcohol-based hand sanitizers may be used if hands appear clean.

Ensure cuts or broken skin are covered with waterproof dressings.

2. Personal Protective Equipment (PPE):

Use disposable gloves for contact with blood, body fluids, mucous membranes, or broken skin. Non-latex options, like nitrile gloves, should be provided for individuals with latex allergies.

Disposable aprons protect clothing from contamination. Impermeable gowns may be necessary in high-risk scenarios.

Masks, face shields, and goggles are essential if splashes to the eyes or mouth are possible. Respiratory viruses like SARS or influenza require fitted FFP3 masks or powered air-purifying respirators during high-risk procedures like intubation.

3. Safe Handling of Sharps:

Avoid direct handling of needles and never re-sheath them.

Immediately discard used sharps in approved containers.

Utilize safety-engineered devices to reduce needlestick injuries.

4. Management of Blood and Body Fluid Spills:

Follow local protocols to clean spills safely, using appropriate PPE and disinfectants (e.g., diluted bleach).

Ensure specimen containers are properly sealed and uncontaminated.

Outbreak Preparedness

ED staff must be prepared for potential outbreaks of severe infectious diseases, such as SARS or pandemic influenza. Effective outbreak management includes:

Utilizing negative-pressure isolation rooms for patients with airborne infections.

Training staff in the correct use of PPE to prevent transmission.

Implementing buddy systems for enhanced safety compliance.

Following established protocols, like Hong Kong's FTOCC criteria (Fever, Travel, Occupation, Clustering, Contact), to assess febrile patients with potential infectious diseases.

Case-Based Analysis: Lessons from SARS

The 2003 SARS outbreak exemplifies the importance of infection control. Improper use of nebulizers and inadequate PPE contributed to widespread transmission among ED staff. Subsequent implementation of strict isolation protocols and PPE training significantly reduced the risk. This case underscores the need for vigilance and preparedness in managing emerging infectious diseases.

Emergency Management at the Scene of a Roadside Incident

Effective emergency management at the scene of a roadside incident requires careful prioritization to ensure the safety of both the rescuers and the victims. Failure to follow fundamental protocols can worsen the situation, delay care, or even endanger rescuers. This guide outlines the essential steps for managing roadside emergencies professionally and efficiently.

Immediate Priorities

1. Ensure Rescuer Safety:

Park your vehicle in a secure location that avoids obstructing traffic, including emergency responders. Use hazard lights and, if available, a warning beacon to alert others to the scene.

Switch off vehicle engines, including those of other involved vehicles.

Eliminate ignition hazards such as smoking or open flames.

2. Notify Emergency Services:

Call emergency services (e.g., 999) and provide the exact location, a summary of the incident, and an estimate of the number of casualties. Identify yourself and share your contact details for follow-up if necessary.

3. Assess Additional Hazards:

In cases involving electricity (e.g., overhead power lines or electrified rail tracks), maintain a safe distance and contact the power company to deactivate the source.

For chemical spills, stay at a safe distance until the fire service declares the area secure. Hazardous chemical vehicles display Hazchem boards with critical safety information.

Chemical Incidents

Hazchem Boards:
These boards provide essential information on evacuation, protective equipment, firefighting protocols, and environmental hazards. They also include a UN identification number and hazard warnings.

White plates indicate non-toxic substances.

Contact the transport company or poison control centers for further advice.

Emergency Resources:
Use tools like the TREM card or CHEMDATA for specific chemical details. Inquire with the National Chemical Information Centre or similar agencies for immediate guidance.

Helicopter Evacuation Protocols

Avoid entering the landing area during helicopter landing or takeoff.

Secure loose objects to prevent hazards caused by rotor winds.

Approach helicopters only with the pilot's permission, maintaining a low posture within their field of vision.

If using a winch, do not touch the cable until it contacts the ground to neutralize static electricity.

Managing Major Incidents

Major incidents, characterized by multiple casualties or complex emergencies, require a coordinated response involving multiple agencies. Hospitals implement Major Incident Plans to streamline resources and responses.

1. Hospital Response:

Inform the emergency department (ED) consultant immediately.

Set up a control center and prepare for patient inflow by clearing wards and notifying staff.

Use triage points staffed by senior personnel to prioritize treatment based on injury severity.

2. Triage and Labelling:

Each patient must be assigned a unique identification number for tracking.

Collect essential details promptly, but prioritize treatment and triage over administrative formalities.

3. Communication:

Avoid overwhelming hospital switchboards by using alternative lines to contact additional staff.

Staff should wear identification badges to ensure roles are clearly recognized.

Incident Site Arrangements

Roles and Responsibilities:

The police oversee overall site management.

The fire service handles immediate risks such as fire or chemical exposure.

Ambulance services manage casualty evacuation.

Medical Teams:

Mobile medical teams, led by a Medical Incident Officer (MIO), coordinate on-site care. These teams must be equipped with protective gear, medical supplies, and clearly defined roles.

The MIO collaborates with the Ambulance Incident Officer (AIO) to distribute casualties appropriately and provide real-time updates to hospitals.

Post-Incident Debriefing

Debriefing ensures that all responders can reflect on the incident, share insights, and address emotional impacts. Counseling may be offered to mitigate stress and prevent long-term psychological effects. Incident reports are essential for refining future response plans and improving preparedness.

For more detailed guidelines, refer to official emergency planning resources such as NHS Emergency Planning Guidance or CBRN decontamination protocols.

Chapter 2
Life-Threatening Emergencies

Anaphylaxis

Overview of anaphylaxis as a severe allergic reaction requiring urgent care.

Treatment Algorithm for Adults with Anaphylaxis: Step-by-step management protocol.

Choking

Identification and management of airway obstruction in adults.

Cardiac Arrest

Recognition and treatment of sudden cardiac arrest.

In-Hospital Resuscitation Algorithm: Structured guidelines for in-hospital cardiac emergencies.

Adult Basic Life Support: Core principles of CPR and resuscitation techniques.

Cardiac Arrest Management: Advanced strategies, including defibrillation and medications.

Advanced Life Support Algorithm: Comprehensive framework for advanced resuscitation.

Notes on Using the Advanced Life Support Algorithm: Practical considerations and tips.

Post-Resuscitation Care

Management strategies following the return of spontaneous circulation.

Central Venous Access

Techniques and considerations for achieving central venous access during emergencies.

Severe Sepsis and Septic Shock

Early recognition and management of life-threatening infections.

Shock
Classification and tailored interventions for different shock states.

Anaphylaxis

Anaphylaxis is a severe, rapid-onset allergic reaction that occurs after exposure to certain allergens. This immune system response can manifest through various mechanisms, such as:

IgE-mediated reactions: These occur when the body reacts to foreign proteins (such as those from insect stings, certain foods, or medications like streptokinase) or protein-hapten conjugates (for example, antibiotics).

Complement-mediated reactions: These are seen in responses to human proteins like immunoglobulin G (IgG) or blood products.

Unclear mechanisms: Conditions like aspirin-induced anaphylaxis or idiopathic anaphylaxis fall under this category.

Regardless of the cause, mast cells and basophils are activated and release various mediators, including histamines, prostaglandins, thromboxanes, platelet-activating factors, and leukotrienes. These compounds trigger the clinical symptoms associated with anaphylaxis. Conditions like angioedema (swelling) caused by ACE inhibitors or hereditary angioedema may present similarly to anaphylaxis. However, hereditary angioedema does not typically involve hives (urticaria) and is treated with C1 esterase inhibitors.

Common Causes of Anaphylaxis

Medications: Including antibiotics, streptokinase, suxamethonium, aspirin, NSAIDs, and IV contrast agents.

Insect stings: From bees or wasps.

Foods: Such as nuts, shellfish, strawberries, and wheat.

Latex.

Clinical Features

The onset and severity of symptoms can vary, but the reaction typically develops within minutes to hours after exposure to the trigger. Early signs may include a sense of impending doom or anxiety. Those on beta-blockers or with underlying heart conditions or asthma may experience more severe symptoms. Anaphylaxis usually affects more than one organ system:

Respiratory: Swelling of the lips, tongue, pharynx, and epiglottis can lead to upper airway obstruction. Lower airway involvement may mimic acute asthma, with symptoms such as shortness of breath, wheezing, chest tightness, hypoxia, and hypercapnia.

Skin: Symptoms include itching (pruritus), redness (erythema), hives (urticaria), and angioedema (swelling).

Cardiovascular: Peripheral vasodilation and increased vascular permeability lead to fluid leakage, resulting in low blood volume, hypotension, and shock. Arrhythmias, ischemic chest pain, and changes on the ECG may also occur.

Gastrointestinal: Nausea, vomiting, diarrhea, and abdominal cramps.

Treatment

1. Remove the Trigger: If an allergen is identified (such as a drug), discontinue its administration. For insect stings, carefully remove the stinger from the skin.

2. Administer Oxygen: Provide 100% oxygen to the patient.

3. Open and Maintain Airway: If swelling in the airway is present, seek immediate specialist assistance. Emergency intubation or a surgical airway may be required in severe cases.

4. Adrenaline (Epinephrine):

Administer 0.5mg (0.5mL of 1:1000 solution) intramuscularly (IM). Repeat every 5 minutes if there is no improvement.

In adults using an auto-injector (e.g., EpiPen®), a 300 mcg dose is usually sufficient. Additional doses may be required.

For patients on tricyclic antidepressants, MAOIs, or beta-blockers, administer half the usual dose of adrenaline.

5. For Severe Cases: In cases of profound shock or life-threatening situations, provide cardiopulmonary resuscitation (CPR) or advanced life support (ALS) as needed. Consider intravenous (IV) adrenaline (1:10,000 or 1:100,000 solution) for experienced clinicians who can gain immediate IV access. If adrenaline is ineffective, glucagon (1-2 mg IM/IV) every 5 minutes may be helpful, especially for patients taking beta-blockers.

6. Bronchodilator Therapy: Administer a nebulized beta-2 agonist (e.g., salbutamol 5mg) with oxygen for bronchospasm. Nebulized ipratropium bromide (500mcg) may be added.

7. IV Fluids: If hypotension persists despite adrenaline, administer IV fluids (1-2L of 0.9% saline) and adjust based on clinical response.

8. Antihistamines: H1 blockers (e.g., chlorphenamine 10–20mg IV) and H2 blockers (e.g., ranitidine 50mg IV) are secondary treatments that may help reduce symptoms. Hydrocortisone (100–200 mg IV) may also be administered to decrease the severity and duration of symptoms.

9. Observation: Patients should be monitored for 4-6 hours after the initial reaction, as prolonged or biphasic reactions may occur.

Reporting and Follow-up: Anaphylactic reactions related to drugs or vaccines should be reported to the Committee on Safety of Medicines. Follow-up may include investigating the cause and possible desensitization. Ensure the patient is informed and a Medic-Alert bracelet is considered.

Treatment Algorithm for Adults

1. Resuscitation:

Airway: Ensure patency, administer high-flow oxygen, and assess breathing.

IV Fluid: Administer an IV fluid challenge: 500–1000mL for adults, 20mL/kg for children (crystalloid).

Chlorphenamine and Hydrocortisone: Administer 10 mg of chlorpheniramine and 200mg of hydrocortisone (IV) for symptomatic relief.

Adrenaline:

IM doses of adrenaline (1:1000 solution) should be administered, repeating after 5 minutes if needed.

Adult dose: 500 micrograms IM (0.5mL).

Children's doses are adjusted based on age.

Monitor: Regularly check pulse oximetry, ECG, and blood pressure.

2. Severe Reactions:

Life-threatening: In cases of airway swelling, difficulty breathing, or circulatory failure, administer CPR/ALS. Consider IV adrenaline only for experienced clinicians.

Monitoring: Continue pulse, ECG, and blood pressure monitoring throughout.

Choking Management

Choking is often caused by airway obstruction while eating, typically indicated by a person clutching their neck. Severe obstruction results in inability to speak or breathe, potentially leading to unconsciousness. Treatment follows these guidelines:

1. Conscious Patient: Administer 5 back blows followed by 5 abdominal thrusts. Encourage the

patient to cough. Continue until the obstruction is cleared or the patient becomes unconscious.

2. Unconscious Patient: Perform CPR immediately.

Cardiac Arrest

Recognition of cardiac arrest is vital. It typically occurs suddenly and without warning, particularly in patients who collapse unexpectedly. If a patient is unconscious and does not have signs of life, initiate CPR without delay. Do not waste time checking for additional signs like pupil response. Begin CPR, and assess the rhythm via ECG if possible.

Team Response: The resuscitation team should act efficiently, performing simultaneous tasks like CPR, defibrillation, and securing an airway. Following the advanced life support (ALS) protocol, the team should ensure minimal interruption to CPR.

Adult Basic Life Support: Airway and Ventilation

In the emergency department (ED), advanced airway management techniques are typically initiated immediately. However, when basic airway management is employed (Fig. 2.4), the following steps should be followed:

Positioning the Patient: Place the patient in a supine position (on their back). To open the airway, perform the head tilt and chin lift maneuver. If cervical spine injury is suspected, use the jaw thrust maneuver instead to avoid exacerbating potential neck trauma.

Clearing the Airway: Remove any visible obstructions from the patient's mouth. However, if the patient wears well-fitting dentures, they should be left in place to help maintain a proper seal during ventilation.

Breathing and Ventilation: Aim for a breath duration of approximately 1 second per ventilation, ensuring that the chest rises with each breath. After each ventilation, maintain the head tilt/chin lift position, remove your mouth from the patient's, and observe the chest to confirm it falls as the air is expelled.

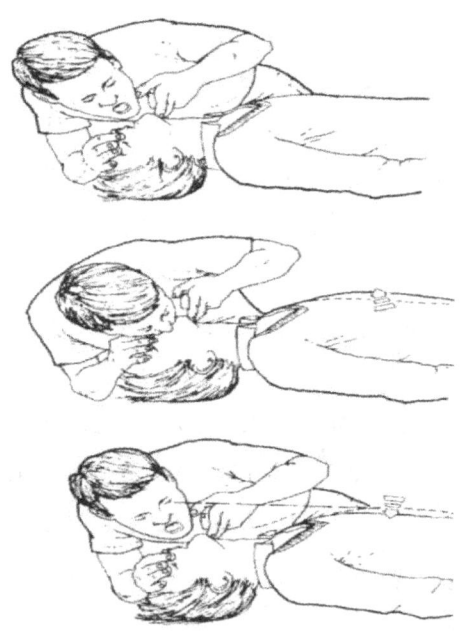

Figure 2-1: Mouth-to-Mouth Ventilation

Technique for Chest Compression

1. Position the heel of one hand on the lower half of the patient's sternum, with the other hand placed on top. Interlock or extend the fingers of both hands to avoid pressure on the ribs.

2. With your arms straight, press down firmly on the sternum, ensuring a depth of 5-6 cm.

3. Allow full recoil of the chest between compressions, and perform at a rate of 100-120 compressions per minute.

4. Maintain an equal time for compression and release phases.

5. Use a 30:2 compression-to-ventilation ratio.

6. Rotate the person performing chest compressions every 2 minutes, ensuring minimal interruption to compressions.

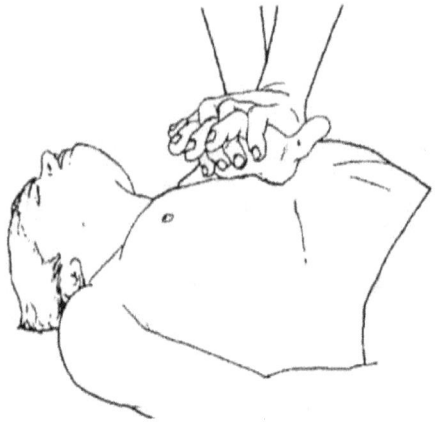

Figure 2-2: Chest compressions

Cardiac Arrest Management: A Comprehensive Approach

Defibrillation: The majority of survivors of cardiac arrest present with ventricular fibrillation (VF) or pulseless ventricular tachycardia (VT). The primary treatment for these rhythms is defibrillation. It is important to note that the likelihood of successful defibrillation decreases significantly over time. In most hospitals, adhesive defibrillator pads have replaced manual paddles. Proper pad placement involves positioning one pad to the right of the upper sternum, just below the clavicle, and the other in the mid-axillary line at the level of the V6 ECG electrode. Avoid placing the pads over the female breast and maintain a distance of at least 15 cm from pacemakers to prevent interference. For biphasic defibrillators, use a shock energy of 150J; for older monophasic defibrillators, use 360J.

Chest compressions should be continuous with minimal interruptions. After a brief pause to assess the rhythm, resume compressions until the defibrillator is charged. Once the shock is delivered, immediately restart CPR with a 30:2 compression-to-ventilation ratio. Continue for 2 minutes before reassessing the rhythm or checking for a pulse. In monitored patients with pulseless VT/VF where defibrillation is not immediately available, a precordial thump may be used. This involves delivering a direct blow to the lower half of the sternum with a tightly clenched fist from a height of 20–30 cm.

Airway Management: Airway management involves securing the airway, providing oxygenation, and ensuring adequate ventilation. Tracheal intubation is considered the gold standard for airway management but should only be attempted by trained personnel. An alternative, the laryngeal mask airway (LMA), is easier to insert and can be a rapid option. Ventilation should aim for 100% oxygen with an inspiratory time of 1 second and a volume sufficient to cause a normal chest rise, at a rate of 10 breaths per minute. When a tracheal tube or LMA is in place, continue ventilation without interrupting chest compressions. End-tidal CO_2 monitoring is essential for confirming correct tracheal tube placement and assessing cardiac output during CPR.

Drug Administration: There is limited evidence supporting the use of drugs in improving survival outcomes during cardiac arrest.

Peripheral venous access is preferred for drug administration due to its ease and speed. If peripheral access is unavailable, the intraosseous route should be considered. It is no longer recommended to administer drugs via the tracheal tube or intracardiac route.

The first drug administered during cardiac arrest is adrenaline. In the case of VF/VT, adrenaline should be given after three shocks. In asystole or pulseless electrical activity (PEA), adrenaline should be given as soon as possible.

Non-Shockable Rhythms: PEA and Asystole
PEA occurs when there is electrical activity on the ECG without an associated pulse, indicating a failure in the heart's pumping mechanism. This can be caused by conditions such as massive myocardial infarction, drug overdose, electrolyte imbalances, tension pneumothorax, or pericardial tamponade. Timely identification and correction of these underlying causes may improve survival outcomes. Asystole, characterized by the absence of electrical

activity in the heart, requires continuous chest compressions and ventilation, with efforts to identify and treat reversible causes.

Resuscitation Duration: The duration of resuscitation attempts should be based on the nature of the event, the elapsed time since onset, and the likelihood of a positive outcome. In cases of persistent VF or pulseless VT, defibrillation attempts should continue. If VF does not respond to defibrillation, consider repositioning the pads or changing the defibrillator. Asystole that does not respond to treatment, especially after prolonged resuscitation (greater than 1 hour), is associated with poor outcomes, although exceptions may occur in cases of hypothermia or drug overdose.

Mechanical CPR Devices: Mechanical CPR devices, such as the "AutoPulse" and "LUCAS" devices, are increasingly used in prolonged resuscitation efforts, particularly in cases involving hypothermia, poisoning, or after fibrinolytic therapy for pulmonary embolism.

These devices provide consistent chest compressions and can free up personnel for other tasks, ensuring quality CPR over long durations.

Reversible Causes of Cardiac Arrest: A structured approach to identifying and treating the reversible causes of cardiac arrest is essential. The "4 H's and 4 T's" represent key factors that should be considered:

4H's: Hypoxia, Hypovolaemia, Hyper/hypokalemia/metabolic disorders, Hypothermia

4T's: Tension pneumothorax, Tamponade, Toxins, Thromboembolic events (e.g., pulmonary embolism)

Advanced Life Support Algorithm: Follow a structured algorithm during cardiac arrest resuscitation:

For shockable rhythms (VF/pulseless VT), initiate defibrillation and high-quality CPR.

For non-shockable rhythms (PEA/asystole), focus on CPR and identify reversible causes.

Administer adrenaline every 3–5 minutes and consider advanced airway management.

Continuously monitor the patient's rhythm and adjust treatment accordingly.

Post-Resuscitation Care: Post-resuscitation care involves ensuring the patient is stabilized and prepared for further treatment. This includes:

Protecting the airway and maintaining ventilation and oxygenation.

Correcting any ongoing issues with blood pressure, cardiac output, or hypoxia.

Monitoring the patient's condition, including using a 12-lead ECG and chest X-ray.

Considering coronary revascularization if the arrest is linked to acute coronary syndrome.

Managing potential complications such as seizures and elevated intracranial pressure (ICP), with appropriate medications and interventions.

Central Venous Access: Indications, Techniques, and Considerations

Indications for Central Venous Access

Central venous access is often necessary for several medical conditions and procedures:

Administration of Emergency Medications: For drugs that need rapid delivery into the bloodstream.

Central Venous Pressure Measurement: To assess blood volume and cardiac function.

IV Fluid Administration: Particularly when peripheral veins are not accessible, such as in cases of collapsed or thrombosed veins. However, for large-volume fluid resuscitation, alternate routes (e.g., femoral vein) are generally preferred.

Transvenous Cardiac Pacing: For controlling heart rhythm during certain emergencies.

Vein Selection for Central Venous Access

The choice of vein for cannulation largely depends on availability, ease of access, and risks involved:

External Jugular Vein (EJV): Easily visible and accessible, often used with standard IV cannulas. However, difficulty arises when attempting to pass a catheter centrally due to valve presence and the vein's angle of entry into the subclavian vein.

Internal Jugular Vein (IJV) and Subclavian Vein: Commonly selected in the emergency department (ED). The internal jugular vein is typically preferred, as cannulation through the subclavian vein carries a higher risk of pneumothorax. The high approach to the IJV is safer and associated with fewer complications. Ultrasound guidance is highly recommended, and using the right side of the neck may minimize the risk of thoracic duct injury. If a chest drain is already in place, cannulation should be performed on the same side.

Femoral Vein: Useful in cases of severe trauma, burns, or when veins are thrombosed, as often seen in patients with substance abuse.

Seldinger Technique for Central Venous Access

The Seldinger technique is the preferred method for central venous access due to its relatively lower complication rate, particularly in preventing pneumothorax. This technique involves the following steps:

1. Needle Insertion: A hollow metal needle is inserted into the vein.

2. Guidewire Insertion: A flexible guidewire is threaded through the needle, after which the needle is removed.

3. Dilator and Cannula Insertion: A tapered dilator and plastic cannula are advanced over the guidewire into the vein.

4. Final Checks: The guidewire and dilator are removed, and the cannula is secured. Venous blood should be freely aspirated to confirm correct placement.

Precautions and Potential Complications

Central venous access carries potential life-threatening risks, including pneumothorax, hemothorax, arterial puncture, damage to the thoracic duct, air embolism, and infection. As such:

Supervision: Expertise is required, particularly when attempting cannulation in hypovolemic, shocked, or agitated patients. If possible, consider deferring the procedure in such cases.

Ultrasound (USS) Guidance: The use of ultrasound reduces complication and failure rates by providing a clear visual of the needle's path and the vein's position relative to surrounding structures. USS can also identify variant anatomy and patency issues.

Contraindications: Conditions such as bleeding disorders or anticoagulant therapy are contraindicated for IJV and subclavian vein access. Additionally, severe pulmonary disease increases the risk of complications, especially with subclavian access.

Procedure Technique

An aseptic technique is crucial to minimize infection risk. Positioning the patient and following proper procedural steps are essential to success:

1. Patient Positioning: If possible, tilt the trolley 10° head-down to enhance venous filling and reduce the risk of air embolism.

2. Post-Procedure Imaging: After successful or attempted cannulation, a chest X-ray should be taken to confirm the cannula's position and check for pneumothorax.

Cannulation Site Descriptions

External Jugular Vein (EJV): The vein runs superficially across the sternocleidomastoid muscle and towards the clavicle. It can be easily seen and palpated. However, inserting a catheter centrally may be challenging due to the valve and angle at which the vein joins the subclavian vein.

Internal Jugular Vein (IJV): Located in the carotid sheath, the IJV runs parallel to the carotid artery. The high approach to the IJV minimizes pneumothorax risks. The procedure involves:

Turning the patient's head away from the side to be cannulated.

Palpating the carotid pulse at the thyroid cartilage level.

Inserting the needle laterally to the artery at a 45° angle, aiming towards the ipsilateral nipple. Successful access is confirmed by aspiration of venous blood.

Subclavian Vein (Infraclavicular Approach): The needle is inserted just below the midclavicular point, advancing horizontally behind the clavicle toward the suprasternal notch. This method typically reaches a depth of 4–6 cm.

Femoral Vein: The needle should be inserted medially to the femoral artery, just below the inguinal ligament, at a 20–30° angle to the skin.

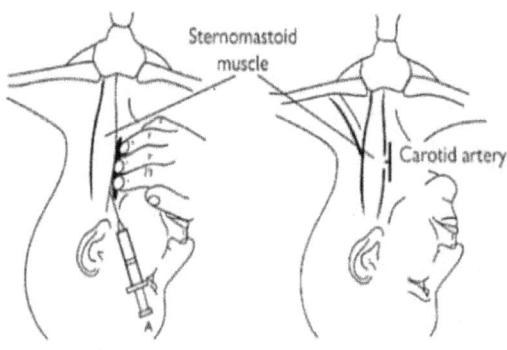

Figure 2-3: Internal jugular cannulation

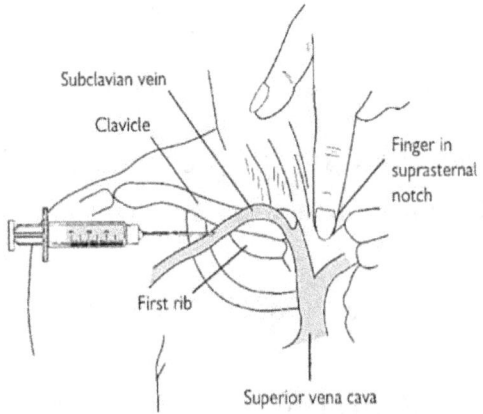

Figure 2-4: Subclavian vein cannulation

Severe Sepsis and Septic Shock

Sepsis occurs as a systemic inflammatory response syndrome (SIRS) due to infection. Severe sepsis is diagnosed when a septic patient shows signs of organ hypoperfusion. Septic shock is diagnosed when patients exhibit hypotension that does not respond to intravenous fluid resuscitation.

Systemic Inflammatory Response Syndrome (SIRS)

SIRS is identified by the presence of at least two of the following clinical signs:

Body temperature > 38°C or < 36°C

Heart rate > 90 beats per minute (bpm)

Respiratory rate > 20 breaths per minute or partial pressure of carbon dioxide ($PaCO_2$) < 4.3 kPa

White blood cell count (WBC) > 12×10^9/L, < 4×10^9/L, or > 10% immature (band) forms

Management of Severe Sepsis

Severe sepsis presents with SIRS and organ hypoperfusion, indicated by symptoms such as a systolic blood pressure (BP) < 90 mmHg or a lactate level > 3 mmol/L. Immediate senior or

ICU consultation is crucial. Key therapeutic goals for managing severely septic patients include:

Central venous pressure (CVP) of 8–12 mmHg

Mean arterial pressure (MAP) > 65 mmHg

Urine output > 0.5 mL/kg/hr

Central venous saturation > 65%

Approach to Management:

1. Obtain senior/ICU assistance immediately.

2. Airway, Breathing, Circulation (ABC):

Provide high-flow oxygen.

Establish secure intravenous (IV) access.

Administer an initial IV fluid bolus (20 mL/kg of 0.9% saline).

Consider early tracheal intubation and invasive positive pressure ventilation (IPPV) if necessary.

3. Identify sources of infection.

4. Check blood glucose (BG) levels and treat hypoglycemia if present.

5. Take blood cultures before starting antibiotics. The antibiotic choice should be based on the suspected infection source (refer to page 60 for details).

6. For patients who remain hypotensive and/or have lactate > 3 mmol/L:

Insert central venous and arterial catheters in an ICU/resuscitation setting.

Use IV noradrenaline to maintain MAP > 65 mmHg.

Administer 500 mL IV boluses of 0.9% saline every 20 minutes to achieve a CVP of 8–12 mmHg (or 12–15 mmHg in mechanically ventilated patients).

Shock

Shock is a clinical condition marked by the inability to adequately perfuse and oxygenate vital organs. It is clinically recognized by the following signs:

Hypotension: Typically, systolic BP < 90 mmHg, though this may vary in young, fit, or hypertensive patients. Tachycardia (heart rate > 100 bpm) is often observed, except in cases with cardiac or neurological causes or in patients taking beta-blockers. In hemorrhagic shock, bradycardia may occur.

Altered consciousness or fainting: This may be due to reduced cerebral perfusion.

Poor peripheral perfusion: Signs include cool, clammy, or pale skin, delayed capillary refill, although early septic shock may present with vasodilation and warm peripheries.

Oliguria: Reduced renal perfusion with urine output < 50 mL/hr.

Tachypnoea: Increased respiratory rate.

Types of Shock

Shock classification is often artificial as mixed etiologies are common. The primary types of shock include:

1. Hypovolemic Shock:

Blood loss: Trauma, gastrointestinal bleeding (hematemesis, melena), ruptured abdominal aortic aneurysm, or ruptured ectopic pregnancy.

Fluid loss/redistribution ("third spacing"): Burns, gastrointestinal losses (vomiting, diarrhea), pancreatitis, sepsis.

2. Cardiogenic Shock:

Primary causes: Myocardial infarction (MI), arrhythmias, valve dysfunction, myocarditis.

Secondary causes: Cardiac tamponade, massive pulmonary embolism (PE), tension pneumothorax.

3. Septic Shock: More common in patients at the extremes of age, those with diabetes, renal or hepatic failure, or those who are immunocompromised (e.g., HIV, malignancy, post-splenectomy, steroid therapy). Fever, rigors, and elevated white cell count may be absent in some patients.

Organisms involved: Include both Gram-positive and Gram-negative bacteria, especially Staphylococcus aureus, Streptococcus pneumoniae, Neisseria , and coliforms, including enterococci and Bacteroides (in intra-abdominal emergencies). In immunocompromised patients, Pseudomonas, viruses, and fungi may also be implicated.

4. Other Types of Shock:

Anaphylactic shock: Refer to page 42.

Neurogenic shock: Refer to page 382.

Other causes: Poisoning (refer to page 183) and Addison's disease (refer to page 155).

Management of Shock

Management and investigation should occur concurrently. Immediate senior assistance is necessary.

1. Address ABC (Airway, Breathing, Circulation).

Provide high-flow oxygen via mask.

Ensure adequate venous access and obtain blood for full blood count (FBC), urea and electrolytes (U&E), glucose, liver function tests (LFTs), lactate, coagulation screen, and blood cultures if necessary.

Monitor vital signs, including pulse, BP, SpO_2, and respiratory rate.

Perform an arterial blood gas (ABG) analysis.

Monitor the ECG and obtain a 12-lead ECG along with a chest X-ray (CXR).

Insert a urinary catheter to monitor urine output hourly.

2. Fluid Resuscitation:

For shock with reduced circulating blood volume, administer 20 mL/kg IV crystalloid

(0.9% saline) bolus. Further fluids, including colloids or blood products, should be given based on clinical response, targeting parameters such as pulse, BP, central venous pressure (CVP), and urine output.

Use caution when administering fluids in cases of cardiogenic shock or a ruptured/dissecting aortic aneurysm.

3. Identify and Treat the Cause of Shock:

Specific treatments depend on the underlying cause and may include:

Laparotomy: For ruptured abdominal aortic aneurysm, trauma (spleen/liver), ruptured ectopic pregnancy, or intra-abdominal sepsis.

Thrombolysis or angioplasty: For myocardial infarction (MI).

Thrombolysis: For pulmonary embolism (PE).

Pericardiocentesis or cardiac surgery: For cardiac tamponade or aortic valve dysfunction.

Antidotes: For certain poisons.

Antibiotics: In sepsis, the antibiotic regimen depends on the suspected cause and local guidelines (e.g., ceftriaxone for meningococcal disease). In cases with no obvious source, empirical combination therapy (e.g., co-amoxiclav, gentamicin, metronidazole) is often recommended. Early microbiological advice is essential, particularly in immunocompromised patients.

Inotropic and vasoactive therapy: As part of goal-directed therapy, assisted ventilation, and invasive monitoring (including arterial and CVP lines) may be required. Specialist ICU assistance should be sought early.

Chapter 3
Comprehensive Management of Critical Medical Conditions

This chapter covers a wide range of topics crucial for medical professionals, specifically focusing on the interpretation of electrocardiograms (ECG) and addressing various cardiovascular, respiratory, neurological, endocrine, and hematological emergencies. Key areas of focus include:

1. Electrocardiogram Interpretation: Critical concepts like the identification of chest pain, angina, acute coronary syndromes, and myocardial infarction through ECG, as well as STEMI treatment and pericarditis. Special attention is given to arrhythmias, including bradyarrhythmias, tachyarrhythmias (both broad and narrow complex), and atrial fibrillation.

2. Hypertensive and Vascular Emergencies: Topics such as aortic dissection, haemoptysis,

oxygen therapy, and the management of dyspnoeic patients are addressed, including challenges like pulmonary oedema and pleural effusion. Also covered are conditions like acute asthma, COPD, and pneumonia.

3. Pulmonary Conditions: Detailed discussion on pulmonary aspiration, spontaneous pneumothorax, deep venous thrombosis, and pulmonary embolism, including their diagnosis and treatment strategies.

4. Gastrointestinal Emergencies: Focus on both upper and lower gastrointestinal bleeding, providing insights on assessment and intervention.

5. Neurological Emergencies: This section emphasizes conditions like stroke, transient ischemic attacks, seizures, and acute confusional states (delirium). Additionally, it explores headache management, subarachnoid hemorrhage, and migraine, including their diagnostic pathways.

6. Endocrine and Metabolic Disorders: Conditions like hypoglycemia, hyperglycemic crises, and sodium imbalances are explored, along with Addisonian crisis, thyrotoxic crisis, and their emergency management strategies.

7. Renal and Urinary Conditions: Discusses urinary tract infections, chronic renal failure, and electrolyte disturbances such as hyperkalemia and hypokalemia.

8. Hematological Emergencies: Covers topics on bleeding disorders, anticoagulant management, blood transfusion, and sickle cell disease, emphasizing timely diagnosis and appropriate interventions.

Electrocardiogram Interpretation

An electrocardiogram (ECG) provides valuable information regarding the heart's electrical activity. To ensure accuracy, the standard recording settings for an ECG are such that each 10 mm deflection corresponds to 1 mV, with a recording speed of 25 mm per second. In this setting, 1 mm represents 0.04 seconds, and each large square on the grid corresponds to 0.2 seconds. A systematic approach should be followed when interpreting the ECG to obtain reliable results.

Heart Rate Calculation

The heart rate can be calculated by dividing 300 by the number of large squares between two consecutive R waves (R–R interval). This simple calculation allows for the rapid determination of the heart rate.

Frontal Plane Axis

The normal frontal plane axis of the heart ranges from −30° to +90° (as shown in Fig. 3.1). For a normal axis, both the QRS complexes in leads I and II should be positive. If the axis deviates beyond this normal range, it may indicate pathological changes:

Left Axis Deviation (LAD): When the axis shifts more negative than −30°, with a positive QRS in lead I and negative in leads II and aVF, it can be associated with conditions such as left anterior hemiblock, inferior myocardial infarction (MI), ventricular tachycardia (VT), or Wolff-Parkinson-White (WPW) syndrome.

Right Axis Deviation (RAD): When the axis exceeds +90°, with a negative QRS in lead I and positive in lead aVF, it is commonly observed in conditions like pulmonary embolism (PE), cor pulmonale, lateral MI, or left posterior hemiblock.

P Wave

The P wave typically lasts less than 0.12 seconds and should be less than 2.5 mm in height. It is most clearly observed in leads II and V1, often used for rhythm monitoring. Certain abnormalities can provide insights into atrial hypertrophy:

A tall, peaked P wave in lead II may indicate right atrial hypertrophy.

A widened or bifid P wave is suggestive of left atrial hypertrophy. In atrial fibrillation (AF), P waves are absent due to disorganized atrial activity.

PR Interval

The PR interval, which represents the time it takes for the electrical impulse to travel from the atria to the ventricles, normally ranges from 0.12 to 0.2 seconds (less than 5 small squares). Changes in the PR interval can indicate specific conditions:

A short PR interval (less than 0.12 seconds) may suggest an accessory pathway (e.g., in WPW syndrome), allowing for faster conduction between the atria and ventricles.

A prolonged PR interval (greater than 0.2 seconds) is indicative of heart block, which can be of varying degrees (first, second, or third degree).

QRS Complex

The QRS complex typically lasts between 0.05 and 0.11 seconds (less than 3 small squares). A prolonged QRS interval may suggest a conduction abnormality, such as:

Right Bundle Branch Block (RBBB): Characterized by an RsR' or M-shaped pattern in lead V1.

Left Bundle Branch Block (LBBB): Demonstrated by a QS or W-shaped pattern in lead V1 and RsR' or M-shape in lead V6. Other causes of a prolonged QRS complex may include tricyclic antidepressant poisoning, hypothermia, ventricular rhythms, and ectopic beats.

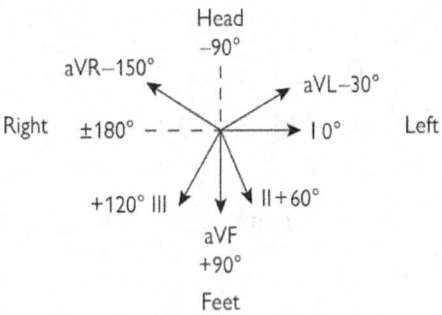

Figure 3-1: Diagram of the ECG Frontal Axis

Amplitude and Key ECG Findings

1. QRS Amplitude: The amplitude of the QRS complex can be an indicator of left ventricular hypertrophy (LVH). Key signs of LVH include:

(S wave in V2 + R wave in V5) > 35 mm

R wave in lead I > 15 mm

R wave in lead aVL > 11 mm

2. Q Waves: Q waves are typically normal in leads III, aVR, and V1. However, they are considered abnormal in other leads if:

The duration is greater than 0.04 seconds or

The amplitude is more than half the height of the subsequent R wave.

3. ST Segment Changes:

Elevation: ST segment elevation can occur in several conditions, such as:

Acute myocardial infarction (MI)

Pericarditis (concave upward)

Ventricular aneurysm

Prinzmetal's angina

Left ventricular hypertrophy (LVH)

Brugada syndrome

Hypertrophic cardiomyopathy

Benign early repolarization

Depression: ST segment depression may indicate:

Ischemia

Digoxin use

LVH with strain

4. QT Interval: The QT interval is measured from the start of the Q wave to the end of the T wave. The corrected QT (QTc) is calculated using the formula:

$$QTc = QT / \sqrt{(R-R \text{ interval})}$$

A normal QTc is < 440 ms.

At a heart rate of 60–100 beats per minute, the QT interval should be less than half the R–R interval.

A prolonged QTc is associated with an increased risk of torsades de pointes, which can be caused by conditions such as:

Acute MI

Hypothermia

Hypocalcemia

Certain drugs (e.g., quinidine, tricyclic antidepressants)

Congenital conditions like Romano-Ward syndrome

5. T Waves:

Inverted T Waves: Inversion of T waves in leads V4-V6 may indicate underlying pathology.

Peaked T Waves: These are often seen in early acute MI or in cases of hyperkalemia.

Flattened T Waves: This can be associated with hypokalemia, sometimes accompanied by prominent U waves.

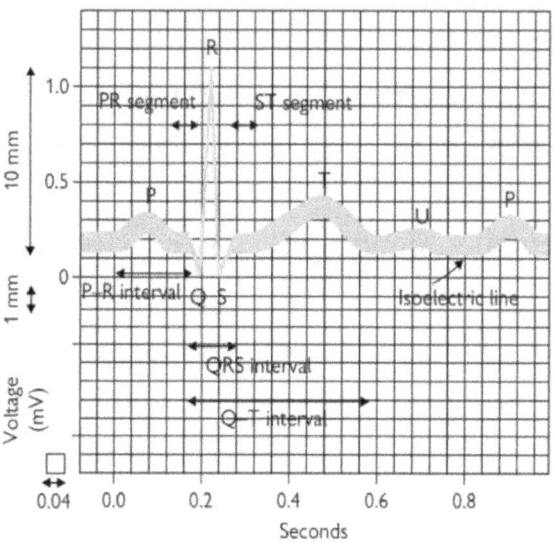

Figure 3-2

Chest Pain: Diagnosis and Management

Introduction Chest pain should always be treated as a potentially life-threatening condition. Immediate triage is essential, with patients requiring urgent evaluation and rapid intervention. Although ischemic heart disease (IHD) is a common diagnosis in middle-aged and elderly patients, it is important to recognize that chest pain can result from a variety of conditions, many of which are also potentially life-threatening.

History: Taking A thorough patient history is critical in determining the cause of chest pain. Key elements to assess include:

Site: Identify if the pain is central, unilateral, or bilateral.

Severity: Assess the intensity of the pain.

Onset and Duration: When did the pain start, and how long has it lasted?

Character: Determine if the pain is described as "stabbing," "tight/gripping," or "dull/aching."

Radiation: Pain radiating to the arms or neck suggests myocardial ischemia.

Precipitating and Relieving Factors: Consider if the pain is triggered or alleviated by exercise, rest, or the use of nitroglycerin (GTN) spray.

Previous Episodes: Any history of similar chest pain should be noted.

In addition, ask about associated symptoms such as breathlessness, nausea, vomiting, sweating, cough, hemoptysis, palpitations, dizziness, or syncope. Be sure to document the patient's past medical history, current medications, and allergies. Accessing old medical records and ECGs can provide valuable insights. If acute coronary syndrome (ACS) is suspected, early consultation with cardiologists is advised.

Examination and Initial Resuscitation A focused clinical examination should assess the Airway, Breathing, and Circulation (ABC). Resuscitation, including the administration of oxygen, venous access, and IV analgesia, should proceed as appropriate. Auscultation of both lung fields is necessary to check for signs of pneumothorax or severe left ventricular failure (LVF). A full physical examination should be conducted to assess for any other underlying conditions.

Investigations The choice of diagnostic tests depends on the presentation, but an ECG and chest X-ray (CXR) are typically required. It is important to note that both of these tests may initially appear normal in cases of myocardial infarction (MI), pulmonary embolism (PE), or aortic dissection. All patients should have continuous ECG monitoring in an area equipped with a defibrillator.

Differential Diagnosis of Chest Pain
(Table 3.1 summarizes common and less common causes of chest pain, with potentially fatal conditions marked with an asterisk.)

Common Causes: Musculoskeletal pain (e.g., costochondritis), acute coronary syndrome

(ACS), pneumonia, oesophagitis, pulmonary embolism (PE).

Less Common Causes: Aortic dissection, herpes zoster, esophageal rupture, pancreatitis, vertebral collapse.

Angina Angina refers to chest discomfort caused by myocardial ischemia, often precipitated by exertion, emotional stress, or cold weather. It occurs when the coronary arteries cannot meet the oxygen demand of the heart muscle (e.g., during exercise, coronary artery spasm, or anemia). The ECG may show ST-segment depression or inversion, which typically resolves after recovery from the ischemic event.

First Presentation of Angina When a patient presents with angina for the first time, there is always concern for the possibility of an MI, especially if the pain lasts longer than 10 minutes (even if relieved by GTN). A normal physical exam, ECG, and cardiac markers do not exclude MI. If there is any doubt, the patient should be admitted, and the case should be discussed with senior medical staff.

Atypical Cardiac Chest Pain It is crucial not to miss cases where patients with acute MI are inadvertently sent home. Chest pain associated with cardiac ischemia may be poorly localized or mimicking musculoskeletal or gastrointestinal issues. Some patients may downplay symptoms to avoid hospitalization. If the clinical history suggests a cardiac cause, particularly with risk factors such as a family history of IHD, hypertension, smoking, or diabetes, the patient should be referred for admission and further investigation. A normal ECG or physical exam should not be reassuring if the clinical history raises concerns. Patients under 30 years old can still experience MI, and sometimes esophageal pain may mimic cardiac pain, improving with GTN.

Acute Coronary Syndromes (ACS) ACS encompasses a range of conditions due to coronary artery plaque rupture, including unstable angina, non-ST-segment elevation myocardial infarction (NSTEMI), and ST-segment elevation myocardial infarction (STEMI). It is important to identify ACS early and begin appropriate treatment.

Management of Unstable Angina and NSTEMI Unstable angina is characterized by worsening chest pain, often at rest, or a new episode of prolonged "crescendo" angina. This condition carries a high risk of progression to MI. In the emergency department (ED), patients with unstable angina or NSTEMI should receive:

Oxygen to maintain oxygen saturation at 94-98%

Continuous cardiac monitoring

IV analgesia (opioid) as needed

Aspirin (300 mg) and Clopidogrel (300 mg)

Low molecular weight heparin (LMWH) for anticoagulation

If pain persists, administer GTN intravenously (provided systolic BP is > 90 mmHg)

Consider Beta-blockers (e.g., atenolol) if no contraindications

Early consultation with cardiology is advised for high-risk patients, especially those with elevated troponin levels or a high TIMI risk score.

TIMI Risk Score The TIMI risk score helps predict the risk of mortality or adverse events based on patient factors (see Table 3.2). Factors include age >65, history of coronary artery disease, recent aspirin use, elevated troponin levels, and ST-segment deviation on ECG.

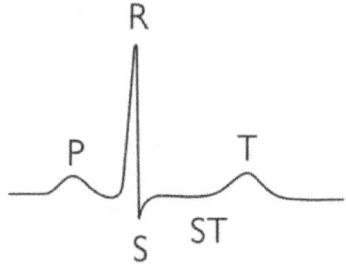

Figure 3-3: Normal lead II

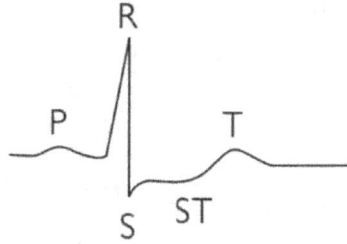

Figure 3-4: Ischaemic changes in lead II

Prinzmetal's Angina

Prinzmetal's Angina, Also known as variant angina, is a type of chest pain that is associated with ST-segment elevation on the electrocardiogram (ECG). This condition is caused by coronary artery vasospasm, which can occur in the absence of any fixed coronary artery blockage or with a pre-existing abnormality. The pain and ST elevation caused by vasospasm may closely resemble an acute myocardial infarction (MI), making it difficult to distinguish between the two conditions. However, unlike an MI, the ST-segment elevation and chest pain in Prinzmetal's angina typically resolve quickly with the administration of glyceryl trinitrate (GTN), providing rapid relief of symptoms. This characteristic helps to differentiate it from an acute MI, which often requires more extensive treatment.

ST-Segment Elevation Myocardial Infarction (STEMI)

Introduction: Ischemic heart disease (IHD) remains the leading cause of death in the Western world. Mortality rates associated with acute myocardial infarction (MI) are estimated at 45%, with a significant portion of these deaths (approximately 70%) occurring before medical assistance is sought. The primary risk factors for MI include smoking, hypertension, advanced age, male gender, diabetes, hyperlipidemia, and a family history of cardiovascular disease.

Pathophysiology of MI: The majority of myocardial infarctions involve the left ventricle and typically result from the sudden occlusion of a coronary artery or one of its branches. This blockage is usually due to thrombosis superimposed on a pre-existing atheromatous plaque. Patients with underlying IHD are at an increased risk of MI, especially when additional stressors such as high levels of carboxyhemoglobin (COHb) from smoking are present. MI may also occur in specific inflammatory conditions such as vasculitis (e.g., cranial arteritis or Kawasaki disease).

Diagnosis of MI: The diagnosis of acute MI is based on the presence of at least two of the following three criteria:

1. A history of typical ischemic chest pain.

2. Evolutionary changes on serial ECGs.

3. A rise in serum cardiac markers.

It is important to note that a normal ECG is seen in 50-60% of patients on initial presentation, and up to 17% may have a completely normal first ECG. Late presentations often do not improve diagnostic accuracy on the ECG.

Clinical Presentation: The classic presentation of MI involves sudden, severe, and constant central chest pain, often radiating to the arms, neck, or jaw. This pain is typically much more intense than typical angina and is unrelieved by nitroglycerin (GTN). Associated symptoms often include sweating, nausea, vomiting, and breathlessness.

However, atypical presentations are common, and a high index of suspicion should be maintained, especially in patients who may misinterpret their symptoms as indigestion (i.e., new-onset "dyspeptic" pain). Approximately one-third of patients may not experience chest pain at all. This is more common in older individuals, females, and those with a history of diabetes or heart failure, and these patients generally have a higher mortality rate. Atypical presentations may include:

Left ventricular failure (LVF),

Collapse or syncope (possibly with injuries like head trauma),

Confusion,

Stroke, or

An incidental ECG finding at a later date.

In assessing a patient with suspected MI, it is crucial to take a thorough medical history, including a background of IHD, hypertension, diabetes, hyperlipidemia, and any contraindications to thrombolysis. Also, ask about drug history, especially the use of substances such as cocaine, which can induce MI.

Physical Examination: Upon examination, the patient may appear pale, sweaty, and distressed. The examination may be normal unless complications such as arrhythmias or LVF are present. Key areas to focus on during the initial examination include:

Checking the pulse, blood pressure, and cardiac rhythm to assess for arrhythmias or signs of cardiogenic shock.

Auscultating the heart for murmurs or the third heart sound.

Listening to the lung fields for signs of LVF, pneumonia, or pneumothorax.

Checking peripheral pulses to rule out conditions like aortic dissection.

Examining the legs for deep vein thrombosis (DVT), which may indicate pulmonary embolism (PE).

Palpating the abdomen for tenderness or masses to exclude alternative diagnoses such as cholecystitis, pancreatitis, perforated peptic ulcers, or ruptured aortic aneurysms.

Investigations: For diagnosing STEMI in the early hours, clinical history and ECG changes are the most reliable indicators. Serum cardiac markers take several hours to rise, so they are less useful in the initial assessment.

Key investigations include:

ECG: Obtain an ECG as soon as possible (ideally within minutes of arrival). In some cases, paramedics may have already recorded a diagnostic ECG. If the initial ECG is normal but suspicion remains high, repeat the ECG every 15 minutes.

Review old medical records for previous ECGs for comparison.

Continuous cardiac monitoring and pulse oximetry are essential.

Monitoring vital signs such as BP and respiratory rate.

Blood tests: Obtain samples for cardiac markers, electrolytes (U&E), glucose, full blood count (FBC), and lipids.

Chest X-ray (CXR) if there is concern about LVF or aortic dissection.

Cardiac Markers: Troponins (cTnT and cTnI) are the most specific and sensitive markers for myocardial injury. However, these markers are only maximally accurate after 12 hours. Elevated troponins can also occur in conditions other than

MI, such as pericarditis, large pulmonary embolism, or sepsis. Renal failure can also impair the clearance of troponins, leading to elevated levels.

Chest Pain Assessment Units: These units are being set up in some emergency departments (EDs) and use a combination of ECGs, ST-segment monitoring, cardiac markers, and exercise testing to assess low-to-moderate risk patients. Patients who do not meet the criteria for STEMI may be discharged within 6-12 hours, but it is crucial to understand that excluding an acute coronary syndrome (ACS) does not fully address the cause of the chest pain.

ECG Changes in MI: When cardiac muscle undergoes infarction, distinct ECG changes evolve over hours, days, and weeks, in a relatively predictable pattern.

1. Hyperacute Changes: Often subtle, these changes can be seen within minutes of infarction:

Prolonged ventricular activation time, as the infarcting myocardium conducts electrical impulses more slowly.

Heightened R wave amplitude, especially in inferior leads in the case of inferior MI.

Upward-sloping ST segment before it becomes elevated.

Tall, widened T waves.

2. Evolving Changes: These changes, especially when combined with a suggestive clinical history, are indicative of MI:

ST elevation: This is the hallmark change and is considered significant if it exceeds 1 mm in two limb leads or 2mm in adjacent chest leads.

Reciprocal ST depression: Seen in the leads opposite to the infarcted area.

Pathological Q waves: Reflecting electrically inert necrotic myocardium.

T-wave inversion: Deeply inverted and symmetrical T waves.

Conduction abnormalities: Left bundle branch block (LBBB) can complicate the interpretation of the ECG. The Sgarbossa criteria help diagnose MI in the presence of LBBB, with specific changes like ST elevation >1mm in leads with a positive QRS, ST depression in V1-V3, or ST elevation >5mm in leads with negative QRS complexes.

3. Chronic Changes: In the months following MI, ECG abnormalities such as ST-segment elevation gradually normalize, but Q waves often persist, indicating the presence of a prior infarction. If a ventricular aneurysm develops, the ST-segment may remain elevated.

Figure 3-5: ECG Changes Following Myocardial Infarction

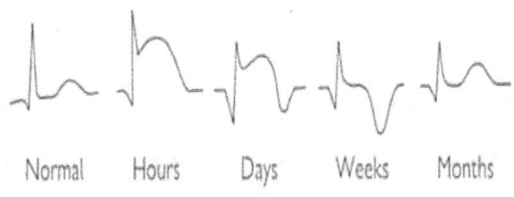

Normal
Hours
Days
Weeks
Months

Figure 3-6: ECG Changes Post-Myocardial Infarction

I
aVR
V_1
V_4
II
aVL
V_2
V_5
III
aVF
V_3
V_6

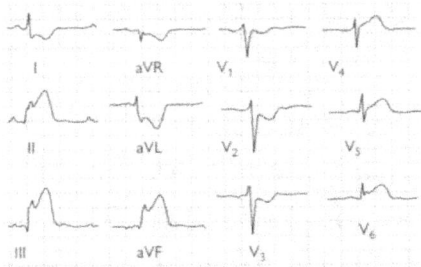

Figure 3-7: Fig. 3.6 Acute inferolateral infarction with 'reciprocal' ST changes in I, aVL, and V 2–V 3

Figure 3-8: Acute anteroseptal infarction with slight reciprocal ST changes in leads III and aVF.

ECG Changes in Myocardial Infarction: Localization and Diagnosis

Localization of Myocardial Infarction (MI)

Myocardial infarction (MI) primarily affects the left ventricle (LV) but can occasionally involve the right ventricle (RV), while the atria are almost never affected. The specific location of the infarction can be determined by identifying the changes seen in different ECG leads.

Posterior Myocardial Infarction

Posterior MI generally occurs in conjunction with inferior or lateral MI. Since conventional ECG leads do not directly capture signals from the posterior heart due to intervening tissues, additional leads (V7-V9) are required for accurate diagnosis. Reciprocal changes in leads V1-V3, such as tall and slightly widened R waves, concave up ST depression, and upright, widened T waves, support the diagnosis of posterior infarction.

Right Ventricular Infarction

Right ventricular infarction often occurs alongside an inferior MI. If ST elevation is present in the inferior leads, ST elevation in lead V1 suggests RV involvement. To confirm the diagnosis, an ECG from lead V4R should be recorded. Recognizing RV infarction is essential for guiding treatment, particularly in managing cardiac failure. IV fluids are needed to maintain adequate filling pressure, and caution is advised when considering the use of nitrates.

Blood Supply to the Heart and Coronary Artery Dominance

The heart's blood supply is primarily provided by the coronary arteries. The left anterior descending artery supplies the anterior and septal areas, while the circumflex artery supplies the anterolateral region. The right coronary artery generally supplies the right ventricle, sinoatrial node, and the inferior wall of the left ventricle. In about 15% of people, the circumflex artery supplies the inferior wall of the left ventricle, indicating left coronary dominance.

In summary, the specific location of myocardial infarction can be identified through characteristic changes in the ECG leads, which provide crucial insights for diagnosis and treatment.

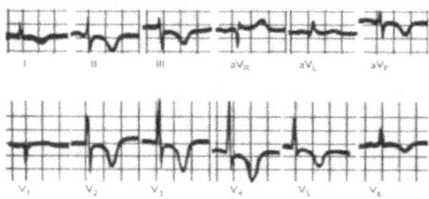

Fig. 3-9: ECG of Subendocardial Infarction

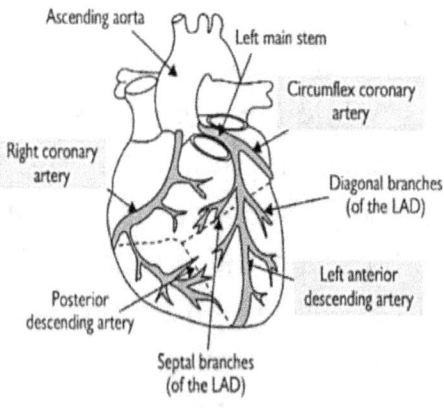

Figure 3-10

STEMI: Treatment Overview

The treatment of ST-segment elevation myocardial infarction (STEMI) requires rapid intervention to minimize myocardial damage. Time is critical, as quicker treatment can prevent irreversible heart muscle injury.

1. Initial Actions

Oxygen should be administered to maintain an oxygen saturation (SpO2) level between 94–98%. A cardiac monitor must be connected immediately.

Secure intravenous (IV) access, and obtain laboratory samples, including U&E, glucose, full blood count (FBC), and cardiac markers.

Administer small doses of IV opioids, titrated based on the patient's pain level.

Ensure the patient receives 300 mg of aspirin and 300 mg of clopidogrel orally to inhibit platelet aggregation.

Contact the cardiology team to arrange for primary percutaneous coronary intervention (PCI) and transport to the catheterization lab.

2. Adjunct Therapy for PCI

If the patient is a candidate for PCI, consider the use of a glycoprotein IIb/IIIa receptor antagonist as per local protocol.

3. Alternative Treatment if PCI is Unavailable

If PCI cannot be performed within 90 minutes, thrombolytic therapy is an alternative. This therapy should not be delayed, particularly in rural settings where it may be administered by ambulance personnel with telemedicine support.

Initiate low-molecular-weight heparin (LMWH), heparin, or fondaparinux as per local guidelines.

4. Pain Management

If the patient continues to experience chest pain, initiate IV nitroglycerin (GTN) infusion (starting at 0.6 mg/hr), adjusting the dosage as needed, as long as the systolic blood pressure is above 90 mmHg.

5. Beta-blockers

Consider administering IV beta-blockers like atenolol (5 mg slowly over 5 minutes, repeat once after 15 minutes) or metoprolol, unless contraindicated (e.g., in cases of uncontrolled heart failure, hypotension, bradycardia, or COPD).

Indications for PCI or Thrombolysis

ST elevation greater than 1 mm in two limb leads, or

ST elevation greater than 2 mm in two or more contiguous chest leads, or

Presence of left bundle branch block (LBBB) with a typical acute MI history.

Primary Angioplasty for STEMI
Primary PCI, which involves coronary angioplasty and stenting, remains the gold standard for STEMI treatment. When performed within 12 hours of symptom onset, PCI significantly reduces both mortality and re-infarction rates. Early intervention yields the best outcomes.

Thrombolysis
If PCI cannot be achieved within 90 minutes, thrombolysis is an option. The effectiveness of thrombolytic therapy diminishes as time from symptom onset increases. However, if PCI is not feasible, thrombolysis should be initiated without delay. For patients presenting more than

12 hours after symptom onset, thrombolysis is no longer beneficial.

Thrombolytic therapy carries risks, including strokes, intracranial hemorrhage, and major bleeds, particularly in older patients, those with hypertension, or those receiving tissue plasminogen activator (tPA). Always explain the potential benefits and risks of thrombolysis to the patient and obtain verbal consent.

Contraindications for Thrombolysis

Head trauma, recent stroke, neurosurgery, or cerebral tumors.

Active gastrointestinal or genitourinary bleeding, or coagulopathies.

Severe hypertension (e.g., systolic BP > 200 mmHg or diastolic BP > 120 mmHg), aortic dissection, or pericarditis.

Pregnancy and certain post-surgical conditions.

Choice of Thrombolytic Agents

Tissue Plasminogen Activator (tPA) is the preferred thrombolytic. The recommended dosage and regimen vary, with common formulations including alteplase, reteplase, and tenecteplase.

Streptokinase, though still used in some areas, has higher allergenic potential and less efficacy after recent streptococcal infections.

Further Management

Arrhythmias are common post-MI, and most do not require treatment unless they lead to life-threatening conditions. Monitor closely for sudden ventricular tachycardia (VT) or fibrillation (VF).

Hypokalemia should be treated if potassium levels fall below 4 mmol/L.

Pulmonary Edema requires standard management protocols, as outlined elsewhere.

Cardiogenic Shock may occur due to severe cardiac dysfunction, necessitating ICU care, echocardiography, and possible surgical intervention if caused by conditions like ventricular septum rupture or aortic dissection.

Pericarditis: Overview and Management
Acute pericarditis, marked by chest pain, fever, and a characteristic pericardial friction rub, may occur alongside or as a complication of myocardial infarction. Its causes include viral infections, tuberculosis, post-cardiac surgery, and certain autoimmune conditions.

Diagnosis relies on clinical findings and ECG changes, which may show concave ST elevation,

PR depression, and potential pericardial effusion.

Management varies with the underlying cause. Viral or idiopathic pericarditis may be treated with NSAIDs, while bacterial causes require antibiotics. Severe cases, such as pericardial effusion or tamponade, may necessitate pericardiocentesis or surgery.

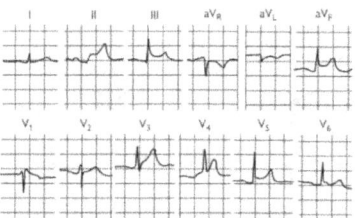

Figure 3-11: ECG of pericarditis.

Bradyarrhythmias: Overview and Case-Based Analysis

Bradycardia refers to a ventricular rate of less than 60 beats per minute in adults and typically indicates abnormalities in the sinoatrial (SA) node or atrioventricular (AV) conduction system. The condition can arise from a range of factors including disease, medications, or physiological changes.

Causes of Bradycardia

Bradycardia is primarily caused by dysfunction or disease of the SA node or AV block, with intraventricular conduction disturbances sometimes leading to more severe AV block. Sinus bradycardia can have several underlying causes:

Physiological: Common in athletes due to enhanced vagal tone.

Pharmacological: Induced by drugs like beta-blockers, which slow the heart rate.

Pathological: Linked to conditions such as hypothyroidism, hypothermia, hypoxia, increased intracranial pressure (iICP), sick sinus syndrome, myocardial infarction (MI), and myocardial ischemia.

Furthermore, bradycardia is observed in up to one-third of patients with hypovolemia, which can occur in conditions like gastrointestinal (GI) bleeding or ectopic pregnancy.

Sick Sinus Syndrome (Sinus Node Disease)

Sick sinus syndrome, often a result of ischemia or degeneration of the SA node, is characterized by sinus pauses (greater than 2 seconds) or sinus arrest. In some cases, escape beats from the junction or other parts of the conduction system may arise. This condition can also lead to tachy-brady syndrome, where both bradycardia and tachycardia occur alternately. Common clinical manifestations include dizziness, syncope, palpitations, and loss of consciousness. Continuous 24-hour ECG monitoring is often necessary to diagnose the arrhythmias associated with this syndrome.

Atrioventricular (AV) Block

AV block refers to delayed or impaired conduction between the atria and ventricles. It can be caused by ischemic heart disease (IHD), certain medications (such as digoxin overdose), or cardiac surgery. AV block is categorized into three degrees:

1. First Degree AV Block: Conduction from the atria to the ventricles occurs with a delay, and the PR interval exceeds 0.2 seconds (five small squares on a standard ECG) but is constant.

2. Second Degree AV Block:

Mobitz Type I (Wenckebach): The PR interval progressively lengthens until a P wave is blocked, meaning it does not conduct to the ventricles.

Mobitz Type II: The PR interval remains constant, but some P waves are blocked and do not result in ventricular conduction. The block may occur regularly (e.g., 3:1) or irregularly.

3. Third Degree (Complete) Heart Block: No atrial impulses are conducted to the ventricles. Depending on the location of the block:

Proximal Block (e.g., AV node): An escape pacemaker in the AV node or the bundle of His may take over, resulting in narrow QRS complexes at a rate of 30-50 beats per minute.

Distal Block: A more distal pacemaker leads to broad, bizarre QRS complexes at a rate of 30-40 beats per minute. If the escape pacemaker ceases to function, ventricular asystole may occur unless another subsidiary pacemaker takes over.

Intraventricular Conduction Disturbances

The intraventricular conduction system starts with the bundle of His, which divides into right and left bundle branches. These branches further subdivide into antero-superior and postero-superior divisions, forming the fascicles. Disturbances in conduction can affect one or more of these fascicles:

Bifascicular Block: Occurs when two out of the three fascicles are blocked, leading to conduction abnormalities.

Right Bundle Branch Block (RBBB) and Left Anterior Hemiblock: This combination results in left axis deviation and an RBBB pattern on the ECG.

RBBB and Left Posterior Hemiblock: Causes right axis deviation along with an RBBB pattern on the ECG.

Trifascicular Block: Involves bifascicular block coupled with a prolonged PR interval, indicating potential progression to complete heart block. It is a precursor to a full AV block.

Clinical Significance

Bradyarrhythmias can significantly impact patient outcomes, particularly if they progress to complete heart block or result in symptomatic episodes like syncope. Effective diagnosis often requires advanced imaging and prolonged ECG monitoring. Treatment strategies may vary depending on the underlying cause, ranging from the adjustment of medications to more invasive interventions like pacing for severe cases.

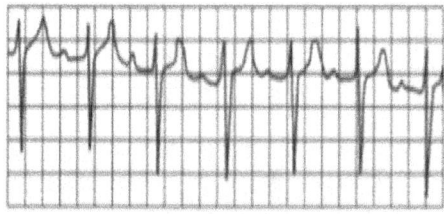

Figure 3-12: ECG of first degree heart block.

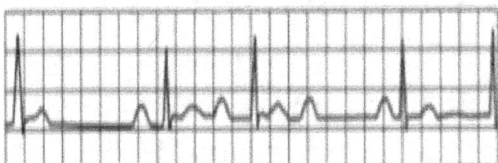

Figure 3-13: ECG of Mobitz type I AV block

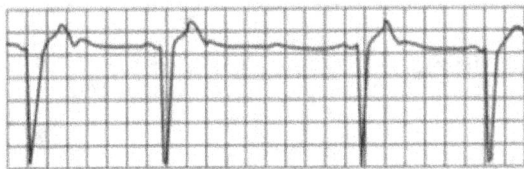

Figure 3-14: ECG of Mobitz type II AV block.

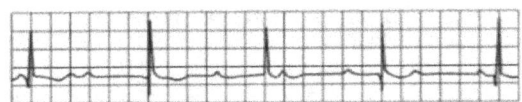

Figure 3-15: ECG of complete AV block.

Treatment of Bradyarrhythmias: A Comprehensive Approach

The management of bradyarrhythmias in emergency settings hinges on two critical factors: the patient's clinical status and the risk of progression to asystole. Early intervention is essential, beginning with supplemental oxygen administration, securing intravenous (IV) access, and adhering to established resuscitation guidelines, such as those provided by the European Resuscitation Council (ERC).

Pharmacological Management

1. Atropine

First-Line Treatment: Atropine is the initial drug of choice for treating bradycardia.

Dosage: Administer 500 mcg IV, repeating as needed up to a maximum total dose of 3 mg.

Limitations: Additional doses beyond 3 mg are generally ineffective and may lead to adverse effects such as psychosis or urinary retention.

2. Adrenaline (Epinephrine)

Indication: Used as a temporary measure in patients awaiting transvenous pacing when external pacing is unavailable.

Dosage and Administration: Administer as a controlled infusion, starting at 2–10 mcg/min, adjusted based on the patient's response. A standard preparation involves dissolving 6 mg of adrenaline in 500 mL of 0.9% saline, infused at a rate of 10–50 mL/hr.

Non-Pharmacological Management

1. External Transcutaneous Pacing

Availability: This option is accessible on most modern defibrillators.

Procedure:

Place adhesive electrodes on the patient's chest and back.

Set the device to the external demand pacing mode at a rate of 70 beats per minute.

Gradually increase the pacing current from zero until electrical capture is confirmed on the monitor.

Clinical Confirmation: Electrical capture should produce a palpable peripheral pulse matching the paced rate and result in an improvement in the patient's condition.

Pain Management: If the patient experiences significant discomfort, administer small doses of IV opioids with or without sedation.

2. Transvenous Cardiac Pacing

Indication: This is the definitive treatment for bradycardia patients at high risk of asystole.

Procedure:

Performed by a skilled practitioner using venous access, typically via the internal jugular or subclavian vein.

In cases where anticoagulation is present or thrombolysis is being considered, the right femoral vein is preferred.

Post-Procedure Care: Obtain a chest X-ray (CXR) to confirm proper placement and rule out complications.

Outcome: A correctly functioning ventricular pacemaker is characterized by pacing spikes on the ECG, followed by widened, atypical QRS complexes.

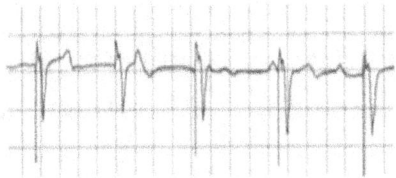

Figure 3-16: Paced rhythm.

Permanent Pacemakers and Implantable Defibrillators: Management and Emergency Considerations

Advancements in implantable devices have significantly improved the management of arrhythmias. However, patients with these devices may occasionally present to the emergency department (ED) with device malfunctions. Prompt and specialized management is essential in such cases.

Immediate Steps in Device Malfunction

1. Seek Specialist Input

Contact a cardiology specialist or electrophysiologist immediately to address the underlying issue and guide further management.

2. Temporary Pacing Support

If the malfunction affects the pacing function, external transcutaneous pacing can serve as a temporary measure until the device issue is resolved.

3. Managing Repeated Defibrillator Firing

In cases where an implantable defibrillator is firing inappropriately or excessively, a specialized magnet may be required to deactivate the device temporarily. This intervention helps prevent unnecessary shocks and stabilizes the patient.

Comprehensive Approach to Bradycardia Management

Management of bradycardia is guided by the presence of symptoms and the risk of cardiac arrest. Below is a detailed algorithm tailored for professional practice based on evidence-based recommendations.

Initial Assessment and Stabilization:

1. Evaluate ABCDE: Assess airway, breathing, circulation, disability, and exposure systematically.

2. Oxygenation and Access: Provide supplemental oxygen if needed, establish intravenous access, and initiate continuous monitoring of vital signs, ECG, blood pressure, and oxygen saturation.

3. 12-Lead ECG: Obtain and review a 12-lead ECG to identify the rhythm and any reversible causes, such as electrolyte disturbances or ischemia.

Decision Tree for Bradycardia:

1. Adverse Features?

Look for shock, syncope, myocardial ischemia, or heart failure.

If adverse features are present, administer atropine 500 mcg IV immediately. Repeat every 3–5 minutes as needed, up to a maximum dose of 3 mg.

2. Evaluate Response to Atropine:

If satisfactory response, continue monitoring and addressing underlying causes.

If no response or signs of instability persist, proceed to interim measures.

Advanced Interventions:

1. Interim Measures:

If atropine fails, consider:

Isoprenaline: Start at 5 mcg/min IV infusion.

Adrenaline: Administer 2–10 mcg/min IV infusion, titrated to response.

Other Drugs: Consider aminophylline, dopamine, or glucagon (for beta-blocker or calcium channel blocker toxicity).

Transcutaneous Pacing: Use external pacing if pharmacological measures are inadequate.

2. Risk of Asystole?

Recent asystole, Mobitz Type II AV block, complete heart block with broad QRS, or ventricular pauses >3 seconds warrant immediate transvenous pacing.

Transvenous Pacing: Insert via the internal jugular or subclavian vein (or femoral vein if anticoagulation or thrombolysis is a concern). Ensure proper positioning with a chest X-ray post-procedure.

Tachyarrhythmia Management Overview

Management of tachyarrhythmias, whether broad or narrow complex, focuses on rapid assessment, rhythm identification, and targeted interventions.

General Approach:

1. Assess ABCDE: Secure airway, provide oxygen, and establish IV access.

2. Monitor Rhythm: Continuous ECG monitoring and 12-lead ECG recording are essential.

3. Identify Reversible Causes: Correct underlying factors such as hypoxia, electrolyte imbalances, or drug toxicity.

Algorithm for Unstable Tachyarrhythmia:

1. Signs of Instability:

Shock, syncope, myocardial ischemia, or heart failure.

Action: Perform synchronized cardioversion.

Atrial Fibrillation or Broad Complex VT: Start at 120–150J (biphasic) or 200J (monophasic). Increase energy if initial attempts fail.

SVT or Atrial Flutter: Start at 70–120J (biphasic) or 100J (monophasic).

2. Post-Cardioversion Measures:

Administer amiodarone 300 mg IV over 20–60 minutes if cardioversion is unsuccessful after three shocks. Follow with a 900 mg infusion over 24 hours.

Broad Complex Tachyarrhythmia:

Assume ventricular tachycardia (VT) until proven otherwise.

VT Indicators:

Age > 60 years, history of ischemic heart disease or cardiomyopathy.

ECG Findings: AV dissociation, capture beats, bizarre QRS morphology (>0.13s), or concordance across precordial leads.

Polymorphic VT (Torsades de Pointes):

Associated with prolonged QT, electrolyte disturbances, or certain medications.

Management:

Administer magnesium sulfate (2g IV over 10 minutes).

Consider overdrive pacing in refractory cases.

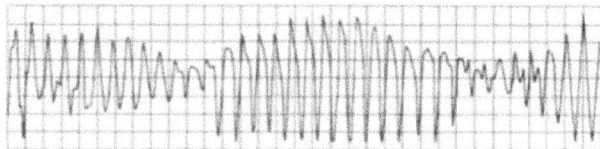

Figure 3-16

Narrow Complex Tachyarrhythmias: Clinical Evaluation and Management

Narrow complex tachyarrhythmias are predominantly of supraventricular origin. The primary rhythms associated with this condition include:

Sinus tachycardia

Paroxysmal atrioventricular reentrant tachycardia (AVRT), often referred to as supraventricular tachycardia (SVT)

Atrial fibrillation (AF) with a rapid ventricular response

Atrial flutter

Atrial tachycardia

Junctional tachycardia

Initial Assessment and Stabilization

1. Oxygenation: Administer oxygen as necessary to maintain adequate oxygen saturation.

2. IV Access: Establish intravenous access promptly.

3. Monitoring: Continuously monitor ECG, blood pressure (BP), and oxygen saturation.

Refer to the tachyarrhythmia management algorithm for guidance (e.g., Fig. 3.17, available at www.resus.org.uk). Begin by determining whether the rhythm is regular or irregular.

For irregular rhythms, such as AF, follow the specific management steps outlined in the algorithm.

If the ventricular rate is approximately 150 beats per minute, consider atrial flutter with 2:1 block as a likely diagnosis.

Emergency Management for Unstable Patients

For patients presenting with shock, syncope, acute heart failure, or cardiac ischemia, immediate synchronized electrical cardioversion is indicated. While preparing for cardioversion, intravenous (IV) adenosine may be administered if this does not delay the procedure.

Management of Stable Patients

1. Vagal Stimulation:

Perform a Valsalva maneuver, the most effective method for vagal stimulation. Instruct the patient to blow into a 50 mL syringe while supine or with a slight head-down tilt.

If the Valsalva maneuver fails, perform carotid sinus massage on one side only (gently massage in a circular motion lateral to the thyroid cartilage for approximately 15 seconds).

Caution: Avoid carotid sinus massage in patients with a carotid bruit or a history of stroke or transient ischemic attack (TIA), as it may lead to complications.

2. Adenosine Administration:

Adenosine temporarily blocks AV node conduction, effectively terminating reentrant tachycardias. It can also reveal underlying rhythms, such as atrial flutter, by inducing a transient conduction block.

Contraindications: Avoid adenosine in patients with second-degree or third-degree AV block,

Wolff-Parkinson-White syndrome (WPW), or asthma.

Precautions: Adenosine's effects can be attenuated by theophylline and potentiated by drugs such as dipyridamole, carbamazepine, or in denervated hearts. Seek expert guidance in these scenarios.

Dosing:

Administer 6 mg IV adenosine as a rapid bolus via a large peripheral vein (e.g., antecubital fossa), followed by a saline flush.

If unsuccessful, repeat with 12 mg, then a further 12 mg if necessary, while monitoring the rhythm continuously.

Side Effects: Warn patients of potential transient flushing, chest discomfort, or a sensation of breathlessness during administration.

3. Alternative to Adenosine:

If adenosine is contraindicated, administer IV verapamil (2.5–5 mg over 2 minutes).

Caution: Avoid verapamil in patients with heart failure, hypotension, concurrent beta-blocker use, or WPW syndrome due to the risk of severe adverse effects.

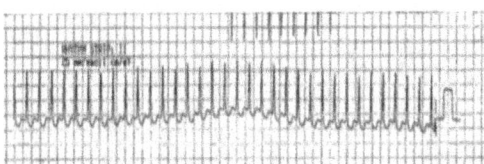

Figure 3-18: Narrow complex tachycardia.

Atrial Fibrillation (AF): Comprehensive Overview and Management

Definition and Clinical Presentation

Atrial fibrillation (AF) is characterized by rapid, irregular, and disorganized atrial electrical activity, resulting in an inconsistent ventricular response. Clinically, AF reduces cardiac output by 10–20%, irrespective of the ventricular rate. While some individuals remain asymptomatic, others may present with symptoms ranging from palpitations to life-threatening complications such as heart failure or angina. Patients with underlying ischemic heart disease (IHD) are at increased risk of myocardial ischemia during episodes of rapid ventricular rates.

Etiology and Risk Factors

Cardiac Causes:

Ischemic heart disease (33%)

Heart failure (24%)

Hypertension (26%)

Valvular heart disease (7%)

Others: sick sinus syndrome, pericarditis, cardiomyopathy, myocarditis, congenital heart disease, post-cardiac surgery

Non-Cardiac Causes:

Sepsis

Pulmonary embolism (PE)

Thyrotoxicosis

Chest trauma

Hypothermia

Electrolyte imbalances (e.g., hypokalemia)

Drug-related triggers (e.g., cocaine, excessive alcohol intake – "holiday heart syndrome")

Special Considerations:

"Holiday heart syndrome" refers to AF caused by binge drinking or alcohol withdrawal in individuals without predisposing conditions, typically resolving within 48 hours after excluding other causes.

Management of AF

Treatment strategies depend on patient stability and the duration of AF.

1. Hemodynamically Unstable Patients:
For patients with shock, syncope, acute heart failure, or ischemia:

Immediate Electrical Cardioversion: Perform under sedation if feasible.

Chemical Cardioversion Options:

Flecainide (50–150 mg IV): Avoid in patients with structural heart disease.

Amiodarone (300 mg IV): Safer alternative for patients with underlying cardiac disease, though hypotension may occur.

2. Stable Patients:

If symptoms persist >48 hours: Administer anticoagulation (IV or low molecular weight heparin) to mitigate thromboembolic risks before cardioversion.

Rate Control Drugs:

Metoprolol (5 mg IV): Effective for rate control.

Diltiazem (IV form may not be available in some regions).

Digoxin (500 mcg IV): Preferred for patients with concurrent congestive heart failure.

Special Situations

Atrial Fibrillation in Wolff-Parkinson-White (WPW) Syndrome:

Presents as irregular, broad-complex tachycardia due to conduction via an accessory pathway.

Avoid AV-Nodal Blocking Agents: Drugs like digoxin, verapamil, or adenosine may accelerate accessory pathway conduction, risking cardiovascular collapse or ventricular fibrillation. Seek expert consultation.

Atrial Flutter:

Atrial rates often approximate 300 beats/min, with ventricular conduction ratios (e.g., 2:1) determining the QRS rate.

Consult a specialist for optimal management strategies.

Hypertensive Disorders: Emergency Department (ED) Approach

General Principles

Hypertension is often asymptomatic and is a significant risk factor for cardiovascular events and stroke.

Acute management is rarely required unless associated with specific symptoms or complications.

Initial Assessment

1. Patients Without Prior Hypertension History: Arrange GP follow-up.

2. Previously Diagnosed Hypertensives on Treatment: Emphasize follow-up and medication review with the GP.

3. Evidence of End-Organ Damage: Immediate referral to a medical team for evaluation of conditions like left ventricular hypertrophy, retinal damage, or renal impairment.

Specific Clinical Scenarios

Hypertension in Stroke: Avoid aggressive blood pressure reductions without specialist advice.

Pain-Associated Hypertension: Treat the underlying cause (e.g., acute pulmonary edema).

Management Based on Severity

Mild/Moderate Hypertension (Diastolic 100–125 mmHg):

Investigations: Urinalysis, ECG, and blood tests (e.g., U&E).

Asymptomatic patients with normal findings can follow up with their GP. Symptomatic patients or those with abnormal findings should be referred to the medical team.

Severe Hypertension (Diastolic >125 mmHg):

Investigate for hypertensive encephalopathy (symptoms: headache, confusion, retinal changes).

Initiate IV access and conduct tests, including creatinine, glucose, ECG, and imaging if neurological symptoms are present.

Refer to a medical team for expert management to avoid rapid BP reductions, which can cause stroke or myocardial infarction.

Treatment Options:

Oral Antihypertensive Therapy: Atenolol or nifedipine may be appropriate.

IV Infusion Therapy: Use sodium nitroprusside, labetalol, or GTN under continuous BP monitoring in HDU/ICU settings.

Sodium Nitroprusside: Short-acting arteriolar and venous vasodilator.

Labetalol: Preferred in suspected aortic dissection or pheochromocytoma.

Avoid Beta-Blockers in hypertension induced by sympathomimetic drugs (e.g., cocaine), as they may worsen hypertension through unopposed alpha-adrenergic activity.

Hypertension in Pregnancy

Pre-Eclampsia/Eclampsia: Diagnosed with hypertension (>140/90 mmHg), proteinuria, and/or edema. Severe cases may involve HELLP syndrome (hemolysis, elevated liver enzymes, low platelets).

Investigate: Urine protein, complete blood count, liver function tests, and coagulation profile.

Eclampsia Management: Seek senior obstetric consultation immediately due to significant maternal and fetal risks.

Aortic Dissection: Clinical Insights and Management

Overview

Aortic dissection is a life-threatening condition often presenting in hypertensive individuals with abrupt, intense chest or back pain. It requires immediate recognition and intervention to prevent severe complications.

Pathophysiology

Aortic dissection occurs due to a longitudinal tear in the aortic media, allowing blood to infiltrate and split the layers. The dissection can extend:

1. Proximally: Potentially causing aortic regurgitation, coronary artery obstruction, or cardiac tamponade.

2. Distally: Affecting branches of the aorta, leading to ischemic complications.

3. Rupture: Either reentering the lumen or externally into structures like the mediastinum, which can result in exsanguination.

Key risk factors include hypertension (present in >70% of cases), bicuspid aortic valve, Marfan syndrome, and Ehlers-Danlos syndrome. Post-surgical or procedural cases account for up to 20%.

Dissections are classified using the Stanford system:

Type A: Involves the ascending aorta.

Type B: Spares the ascending aorta.

Mortality rates are high, with approximately 35% for type A and 15% for type B.

Clinical Presentation

Aortic dissection often mimics myocardial infarction, demanding a high index of suspicion. Key features include:

Sudden onset of sharp, tearing chest or back pain, often at maximum intensity from the beginning.

Pain migration, indicating progression of the dissection.

Syncope in 8–10% of cases, occasionally without accompanying pain.

Neurological deficits associated with ischemia in affected vascular territories.

Physical Examination

Patients frequently appear distressed with unrelenting pain. Diagnostic clues include:

Aortic regurgitation murmur (30%).

Asymmetric or absent peripheral pulses (15–20%).

Hypertension or, conversely, hypotension with tamponade or neurological deficits.

Diagnostic Evaluation

1. Laboratory Tests: Blood work including FBC, coagulation, U&E, and cross-matching.

2. Imaging:

Chest X-ray abnormalities (seen in 87%): widened mediastinum, "double-knuckle" aorta, left pleural effusion, or tracheal deviation.

ECG findings: Often normal but may indicate myocardial ischemia or left ventricular hypertrophy.

Advanced imaging (e.g., CT angiography or transesophageal echocardiography) confirms the diagnosis.

Management

Immediate intervention is crucial. Initial steps include:

1. Stabilization:

Oxygen supplementation as needed.

Pain management with intravenous morphine.

Blood pressure control, typically with IV labetalol, under specialist guidance.

2. Specialist Involvement:

Early involvement of cardiothoracic surgery and cardiology teams.

3. Definitive Treatment:

Type A Dissections: Surgical repair.

Type B Dissections: Medical management unless complications arise.

Arterial Blood Gas Analysis: A Comprehensive Overview

Clinical Utility of Arterial Blood Gas (ABG) Sampling

ABG analysis is a vital diagnostic tool for evaluating patients experiencing respiratory distress, sepsis, diabetic ketoacidosis, critical illness, or toxic ingestion. This test facilitates the rapid measurement of key parameters such as blood pH, bicarbonate (HCO_3^-), oxygen (O_2), and carbon dioxide (CO_2). Modern blood gas analyzers often provide additional metrics, including glucose, potassium (K^+), hemoglobin (Hb), and lactate levels, allowing concurrent evaluation of anemia, hyperkalemia, and hypoglycemia.

Assessment of Respiratory Function

Arterial sampling is particularly useful in patients with low oxygen saturation (SpO_2) or known pulmonary conditions, especially when they are receiving supplemental oxygen. Initial sampling, when feasible, should be conducted while the patient breathes room air; otherwise, the inspired oxygen concentration must be documented. Key findings include:

Hypoxia: Partial pressure of oxygen (pO_2) < 10.6 kPa on room air.

Hypercarbia: Partial pressure of carbon dioxide (pCO_2) > 6.0 kPa.

Bicarbonate Retention: HCO_3^- > 28 mmol/L.

Acidosis: pH < 7.35.

Differentiation of Respiratory Failures

1. Type I Respiratory Failure:

Characterized by hypoxia with normal or low pCO_2.

2. Type II Respiratory Failure:

Characterized by hypoxia with elevated pCO_2 and often increased HCO_3^-.

These patients may experience life-threatening respiratory compromise with high-concentration oxygen. SpO_2 should be maintained at 88–92%, with ABG reassessed in 30 minutes.

Acute vs. Chronic Type II Respiratory Failure

Chronic Type II failure exhibits increased pCO_2 and HCO_3^- as a compensatory mechanism by the kidneys over several days, buffering respiratory acidosis.

Acute failure presents with respiratory acidosis (pCO_2 elevation and pH < 7.35) due to the inability to eliminate CO_2, often necessitating ventilatory support.

Additional Considerations

Venous blood sampling is reliable for assessing K^+, lactate, glucose, HCO_3^-, Hb, and carboxyhemoglobin (COHb). A normal venous pCO_2 effectively excludes hypercarbia.

Interpretation of ABG Results

1. Base Excess:

Calculated from HCO_3^- and pH.

Values < –2 mmol/L indicate metabolic acidosis, while values > 2 mmol/L suggest metabolic alkalosis.

2. Metabolic Acidosis:

Typical findings: pH < 7.35, HCO_3^- < 24 mmol/L, and base excess < –2 mmol/L.

Common causes include increased acid production (e.g., lactic acidosis, ketoacidosis, toxic ingestion), impaired acid elimination (renal failure), or bicarbonate loss (e.g., diarrhea, fistulas).

3. Anion Gap:

Formula: $(Na^+ + K^+) - (Cl^- + HCO_3^-)$. Normal range: 12–16 mmol/L.

High anion gap metabolic acidosis is often due to lactic acidosis or ketoacidosis.

Normal anion gap acidosis is associated with conditions such as chronic diarrhea and renal tubular acidosis.

4. Osmolal Gap:

Calculated osmolarity: $(2 \times Na^+)$ + urea + glucose (mmol/L).

Normal osmolal gap: < 10 mOsm/kg. Elevated values suggest toxic ingestions (e.g., methanol, ethylene glycol).

Cardiogenic Pulmonary Edema: Pathophysiology and Management

Etiology:

Cardiogenic pulmonary edema results from increased left ventricular end-diastolic pressure, leading to elevated pulmonary capillary hydrostatic pressure. Common causes include myocardial infarction, arrhythmias, valvular diseases, and cardiomyopathies.

Clinical Presentation:

Symptoms include severe dyspnea, tachycardia, tachypnea, cyanosis, and pink frothy sputum. Signs such as elevated jugular venous pressure (JVP), fine inspiratory crackles, and peripheral coolness are characteristic.

Diagnostic Workup:

Essential investigations include ECG, ABG (if $SpO_2 < 94\%$), chest X-ray, and laboratory tests for electrolytes, glucose, hemoglobin, and cardiac biomarkers.

Initial Management:

1. Clear the airway and position the patient upright.

2. Administer high-flow oxygen via a tight-fitting mask.

3. Provide sublingual glyceryl trinitrate (GTN) and intravenous furosemide.

4. Address underlying causes, including arrhythmias or myocardial infarction.

5. Consider advanced interventions such as non-invasive ventilation or ICU referral for inotropic support in refractory cases.

Non-Cardiogenic Pulmonary Edema

Unlike cardiogenic pulmonary edema, non-cardiogenic forms arise from increased capillary permeability, decreased plasma oncotic pressure, or elevated lymphatic pressure. Common causes include acute respiratory distress syndrome (ARDS), infections, and toxic exposures.

Assessment and Management of Acute Asthma

For the assessment and management of acute asthma in adults, follow the British Thoracic Society (BTS) guidelines. These guidelines emphasize the importance of addressing factors contributing to asthma-related mortality, particularly in patients with severe asthma who have adverse psychosocial factors such as psychiatric illness, substance abuse, or unemployment, which increase mortality risk.

Initial Assessment

Measure Peak Expiratory Flow Rate (PEFR) and compare it with the predicted or personal best value. PEFR serves as an immediate triage tool; however, patients with life-threatening asthma may be unable to perform this test due to severe dyspnea.

Assess the severity of acute asthma based on clinical features, PEFR, and pulse oximetry.

Severity Classification

Moderate Asthma Exacerbation

Symptoms are progressively worsening.

PEFR is 50–75% of the predicted or best value.

No signs of acute severe asthma.

Acute Severe Asthma

Presence of any one of the following:

Difficulty completing sentences in one breath.

Respiratory rate ≥25 breaths per minute.

Heart rate ≥110 beats per minute.

PEFR is 33–50% of the predicted or best value.

Life-Threatening Asthma

Severe asthma with any one of the following signs:

Cyanosis, exhaustion, confusion, or coma.

Weak respiratory effort or "silent chest."

SpO_2 < 92%.

Bradycardia, arrhythmias, or hypotension.

pO_2 < 8 kPa.

Normal pCO_2 (4.6–6.0 kPa).

PEFR < 33% of the predicted or best value.

Near-Fatal Asthma

Elevated pCO_2 and/or the need for mechanical ventilation with increased inflation pressures.

Additional Investigations

Perform an arterial blood gas (ABG) test if SpO_2 is below 92% or if there are signs of life-threatening asthma.

Obtain a chest X-ray (CXR) without delaying treatment if:

Pneumomediastinum or pneumothorax is suspected.

Consolidation is suspected.

The patient presents with life-threatening asthma.

There is inadequate response to treatment.

Ventilation support is required.

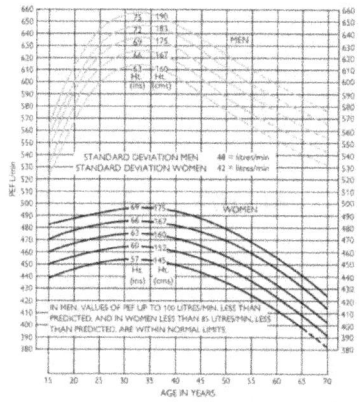

Figure 3-19: Peak Expiratory Flow Rates in Healthy Adults

Management of Acute Asthma: A Detailed Overview

Initial Treatment

Follow the guidelines set by the British Thoracic Society (BTS) and Scottish Intercollegiate Guidelines Network (SIGN), summarized below for clarity and effectiveness:

1. Oxygen Administration:

Administer high-flow oxygen to ensure adequate oxygenation.

2. Patient Positioning:

Place the patient on a trolley with side rails raised, encouraging them to sit upright. This allows the use of accessory muscles, like the pectorals, to facilitate breathing.

3. Initial Treatment and Monitoring:

If the patient is unable to speak, initiate treatment immediately while preparing for possible advanced interventions, including intubation and ventilation. Ensure senior medical staff (ED and ICU) are alerted for immediate assistance.

Assess for signs of pneumothorax by examining the trachea and chest.

4. Medication:

Administer a high-dose nebulized $\beta2$ agonist such as salbutamol (5 mg) or terbutaline (10 mg), or alternatively, deliver 10 puffs of salbutamol via a spacer and mask. For patients showing poor initial response, consider continuous nebulization.

Administer corticosteroids such as 40–50 mg of oral prednisolone or 100 mg IV hydrocortisone.

Add nebulized ipratropium bromide (500 mcg) if the asthma is severe or if the response to $\beta2$ agonists is inadequate.

For severe or life-threatening asthma, and after consultation with senior medical staff, consider a single dose of IV magnesium sulfate (1.2–2 g over 20 minutes).

In refractory cases, consider IV aminophylline, but only after consulting senior medical staff. A typical loading dose is 5 mg/kg IV over 20 minutes, adjusting based on the patient's previous theophylline levels.

In severe cases, IV salbutamol can be considered; consult senior staff for dosing instructions.

5. Additional Considerations:

Dehydration may occur if the patient is unable to talk or drink. Hydration should be considered.

Avoid routine antibiotic use unless there is evidence of infection.

Repeat arterial blood gas (ABG) assessment within the hour.

Monitor for hypokalemia, which can be induced or exacerbated by β2 agonists and steroid therapy.

Criteria for Admission

Patients requiring admission typically present with:

Life-threatening or near-fatal asthma exacerbations.

Severe attacks that persist despite initial treatment.

Discharge Management

Discharge is considered when a patient's peak flow is over 75% of their best or predicted value 1 hour after initial treatment. If the peak expiratory flow rate (PEFR) is less than 50%, a course of oral prednisolone (40–50 mg for 5 days) is recommended. Patients should also be given an adequate supply of inhalers. Ideally, a review by an asthma liaison nurse should occur before discharge, covering inhaler technique and peak expiratory flow monitoring. A follow-up appointment should be scheduled within 2 days, and the discharge summary should be sent to the GP. Patients should be advised to return to the hospital if symptoms worsen.

Referral to Intensive Care Unit (ICU)

Refer patients requiring ventilatory support or those with severe, life-threatening asthma not responding to therapy. Indications for ICU transfer include:

Severe drowsiness or confusion.

Extreme exhaustion with feeble respiration.

Coma or respiratory arrest.

Persistent or worsening hypoxia and hypercapnia.

ABG showing reduced pH.

Deteriorating peak flow.

Cardiac Arrest in Acute Asthma

Cardiac arrest in acute asthma typically results in pulseless electrical activity (PEA), often linked to prolonged hypoxia, arrhythmias due to hypoxia, or tension pneumothorax. Advanced life support should be administered according to established protocols. Early tracheal intubation is crucial to minimize the risks of high inflation pressures and gastric insufflation in the absence of a secure airway.

Chronic Obstructive Pulmonary Disease (COPD)

COPD is defined by chronic airflow limitation primarily due to the obstruction of expiratory airflow, caused by factors such as chronic inflammation, bronchospasm, and airway remodeling, often as a result of smoking. Other causes include chronic asthma, α-1 antitrypsin deficiency, and recurrent respiratory infections such as bronchiectasis.

History and Symptoms

Common complaints include exertional dyspnea, chronic cough, and sputum production. Key elements of the patient's history should include:

Current treatments such as inhalers, steroids, nebulizers, and oxygen therapy.

A history of previous hospitalizations and associated comorbidities.

Exercise tolerance—assessing how far the patient can walk without stopping or how many stairs they can climb.

Recent exacerbations and any changes in sputum color or volume.

Examination

Physical examination often reveals:

Dyspnea, tachypnea, and use of accessory muscles.

Hyperinflation (barrel chest) and wheezing or crackles.

Cyanosis and signs of right heart failure (cor pulmonale) in advanced disease.

Evidence of hypercapnia may include tremor, bounding pulses, confusion, or drowsiness.

Examine for other conditions that may complicate the presentation of COPD, such as asthma, pulmonary edema, or pneumothorax.

Investigations

Basic vital signs: SpO2, respiratory rate, pulse rate, blood pressure, temperature, and peak flow.

Chest X-ray: To check for pneumothorax, hyperinflation, bullae, or pneumonia.

ECG and ABG (or capillary blood gas) to monitor respiratory status and guide oxygen therapy.

Blood tests: FBC, U&E, glucose, and theophylline levels. If pneumonia is suspected, blood cultures, CRP, and pneumococcal antigen testing are also recommended. Sputum cultures should be obtained if the sputum is purulent.

Treatment

1. Oxygen Therapy:

The aim is to maintain an SpO2 of 88–92%. For patients with known COPD and a history of hypercapnic respiratory failure, provide oxygen at 28% via a Venturi mask.

2. Bronchodilators and Steroids:

Administer nebulized salbutamol (5 mg) or terbutaline (5–10 mg).

Consider adding nebulized ipratropium (500 mcg).

Oral steroids such as prednisolone (30 mg) or IV hydrocortisone (100 mg) should be given.

3. Antibiotics:

If purulent sputum is present or pneumonia is suspected, antibiotics such as amoxicillin, tetracycline, or clarithromycin should be started.

4. Additional Medications:

If nebulized bronchodilators are ineffective, consider IV aminophylline or salbutamol.

Non-Invasive Ventilation (NIV)

Non-invasive ventilation (NIV), particularly BiPAP, is standard for managing hypercapnic respiratory failure during COPD exacerbations. NIV has been shown to improve blood gas parameters, reduce intubation rates, and shorten hospital stays. However, it is contraindicated in cases of coma, vomiting, apnea, or cardiac arrest, and should not be used if there is a pneumothorax.

BiPAP settings should start with an inspiratory positive airway pressure (IPAP) of 10 cmH2O and an expiratory positive airway pressure

(EPAP) of 5 cmH2O. These can be adjusted depending on the patient's response. CPAP can also be used for mild cases but is generally less effective in treating severe COPD exacerbations.

Pneumonia

Pneumonia is a common cause of infection, presenting with symptoms such as cough, fever, and breathlessness. It is typically associated with abnormal chest X-ray findings, although some cases, like Pneumocystis pneumonia, may not show significant radiological changes.

Causes

Bacterial: The most common cause is Streptococcus pneumoniae, with other causes including Mycoplasma pneumoniae, Haemophilus influenzae, and Legionella. Consider TB in patients at risk, including those with poor social circumstances or immunocompromised states.

Viral: Includes influenza, respiratory syncytial virus (RSV), and occasionally varicella.

Other: Rickettsial infections (e.g., Coxiella) are rare but possible.

Symptoms

Common symptoms include fever, cough, and sputum production, with potential additional signs such as pleuritic chest pain, hemoptysis, and myalgia. In some cases, particularly with Mycoplasma pneumonia, symptoms may present with less prominent chest signs.

Treatment

Antibiotic therapy should be guided by the pathogen and severity of the pneumonia, with options including amoxicillin, tetracycline, or clarithromycin. Supportive treatment involves fluids, oxygen, and occasionally steroids or antivirals if viral pneumonia is suspected.

Spontaneous Pneumothorax: Detailed Overview

Definition and Types: Spontaneous pneumothorax (SP) is the presence of air in the pleural space without a clear external cause. It can be classified into two types:

Primary Spontaneous Pneumothorax (PSP): Occurs in individuals with no underlying lung disease, typically affecting young, healthy individuals, especially those with tall, thin body types.

Secondary Spontaneous Pneumothorax (SSP): Arises in individuals with pre-existing lung conditions such as chronic obstructive pulmonary disease (COPD), tuberculosis, asthma, bronchial carcinoma, Marfan's syndrome, cystic fibrosis, or following esophageal rupture.

Clinical Presentation: The most common presenting symptoms of spontaneous pneumothorax include:

Unilateral pleuritic chest pain

Dyspnea (shortness of breath)

On physical examination, signs may include:

Tachypnea (rapid breathing)

Tachycardia (elevated heart rate)

Hyper-resonance on percussion over the affected area

Decreased or absent breath sounds on the affected side

Severe symptoms, such as inability to speak, gasping, and low oxygen saturation (SpO_2), suggest a tension pneumothorax and require urgent intervention. Signs of tension pneumothorax include:

Tracheal deviation

Hypotension

Tachycardia

Tachypnea

If these signs are present, immediate decompression with a needle thoracostomy should be performed.

Diagnosis and Investigation:

Pulse, oxygen saturation (SpO_2), blood pressure (BP), and temperature should be monitored in all patients.

High-flow oxygen therapy is administered, particularly in patients with underlying COPD, aiming for an SpO$_2$ of 90–92%.

An arterial blood gas (ABG) analysis can help assess oxygenation status, especially in patients with chronic lung diseases.

Chest X-ray (CXR) is the primary imaging technique. Key points to assess on CXR include:

Displacement of the pleural line

Differentiating the scapular edge from the lung edge

Identifying emphysematous bullae in patients with COPD, which may mimic a pneumothorax

CT scan may be used in stable patients for further assessment, particularly to evaluate bullous lung disease, but is not routinely used for initial diagnosis.

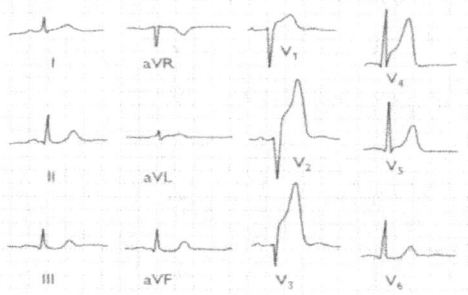

Treatment Approaches:

Management is symptom-dependent:

Needle aspiration is the first line for PSP, performed with a 16G cannula to aspirate air, with a target volume of up to 2.5L.

If needle aspiration is unsuccessful, chest drain insertion via a technique is indicated.

For symptomatic SSP, chest drain insertion is required, along with admission.

Patients without symptoms or with small pneumothoraces (less than 2cm) may be observed with high-flow oxygen therapy and follow-up.

Aspiration and Drainage Techniques:

1. Aspiration:

Confirm the side of the pneumothorax and sit the patient upright.

Administer local anesthesia (1% lidocaine).

Insert a 16G IV cannula into the 2nd intercostal space in the midclavicular line or alternatively, in the 5th intercostal space in the anterior axillary line.

Attach a three-way tap and use a 50mL syringe to aspirate air. Continue until the patient coughs or a maximum of 2.5L of air is removed.

2. Chest Drain Insertion:

Confirm the side of the pneumothorax and ensure the patient is comfortable with adequate analgesia.

Infiltrate 1% lidocaine in the 5th intercostal space at the anterior axillary line.

Use an introducer needle to access the pleural space and pass a guidewire.

Make a small incision, insert a dilator, and pass the chest drain over the guidewire.

Secure the drain with sutures and connect it to an underwater seal. Monitor for bubbling and arrange for a follow-up CXR.

Discharge Criteria and Follow-Up:

Patients with small PSP, minimal symptoms, and no significant breathlessness may be discharged with instructions to seek immediate medical attention if symptoms worsen. A follow-up appointment with a respiratory specialist should be arranged within a week.

Management of Deep Venous Thrombosis (DVT) and Pulmonary Embolism (PE):

Pathophysiology: DVT and PE represent different manifestations of the same disease process, where abnormal clotting in the veins leads to thrombus formation. When a clot dislodges from the vein, it can travel to the lungs, resulting in a pulmonary embolism. Untreated DVT can result in a 1-2% mortality rate due to PE, while approximately 50% of patients with DVT develop post-thrombotic syndrome, which causes long-term pain and swelling.

Risk Factors for DVT:

Recent surgery (especially orthopedic, abdominal, spinal, and obstetric surgeries)

Recent hospitalization

Active cancer

Immobility, such as from fractures or prolonged bed rest

Pregnancy, pelvic masses, and sepsis

History of previous DVT/PE

Thrombophilia or family history of venous thromboembolism

Clinical Features:

Classic symptoms of DVT include leg pain, swelling, warmth, and tenderness, but these signs are not always present, and a small thrombus may be asymptomatic.

Clinical examination is essential but insufficient to rule out DVT. If DVT is suspected, further investigation is necessary.

Pulmonary embolism (PE) symptoms, such as tachycardia, hypoxia, increased respiratory rate, and breathlessness, may suggest the need for a PE investigation.

Diagnosis:

Wells Score: A clinical prediction rule used to assess the probability of DVT. A score of 3 or more indicates a high likelihood of DVT and warrants further investigation.

If the Wells score suggests DVT is unlikely, a D-dimer test can help rule out the condition.

Ultrasound is the gold standard for diagnosing DVT. For patients with a "likely" Wells score, ultrasound is required to confirm the diagnosis.

Management of DVT:

For patients with a high likelihood of DVT, initiate low-molecular-weight heparin (LMWH) until ultrasound results are available.

If DVT is confirmed, continue anticoagulation therapy with LMWH or oral anticoagulants (e.g., warfarin or direct oral anticoagulants).

Upper limb DVT is most commonly seen in patients with central or long-line catheters. If suspected, perform an ultrasound or CT scan.

Differential Diagnosis for DVT:

Conditions like muscular tear, Baker's cyst rupture, and cellulitis can mimic DVT. These should be considered in the differential diagnosis if DVT is suspected.

Management of Superficial Thrombophlebitis:

Superficial thrombophlebitis presents as a painful, tender area in the skin along a superficial vein. It may coexist with DVT. Management typically involves NSAIDs and symptomatic relief. If there's any uncertainty about DVT presence, follow the DVT diagnostic protocol.

Pulmonary Embolism Investigation:

If PE is suspected, initiate investigation with imaging (CT pulmonary angiography) and laboratory tests. Blood gasses, FBC, and U&Es are essential for assessing the patient's status.

Upper Gastrointestinal Bleeding (UGIB)

Causes of Upper GI Bleeding

Common Causes:

Peptic Ulcers: Often due to Helicobacter pylori infection or NSAID use.

Mucosal Inflammation: Conditions like esophagitis, gastritis, and duodenitis.

Esophageal Varices: Caused by portal hypertension, often due to liver cirrhosis.

Mallory-Weiss Tear: A tear in the esophagus, often due to severe vomiting.

Gastric Carcinoma: A rare but serious cause of upper GI bleeding.

Coagulation Disorders: Conditions like thrombocytopenia or anticoagulant therapy (e.g., warfarin).

Rare Causes:

Aorto-Enteric Fistula: Occurs after aortic surgery.

Benign Tumors: Such as leiomyomas, carcinoid tumors, or angiomas.

Congenital Disorders: Ehlers-Danlos syndrome, Osler-Weber-Rendu syndrome, pseudoxanthoma.

History

A comprehensive history is crucial while resuscitating the patient. Upper GI bleeding typically presents with hematemesis (vomiting blood) and/or melaena (black, tarry stools). Significant upper GI bleeding may also manifest as fresh PR (per rectum) bleeding.

Key questions include:

Amount and Duration: Ask about the volume and timing of bleeding.

Past History: Inquire about any previous GI bleeding, liver disease, or related conditions.

Associated Symptoms: Abdominal pain, weight loss, or anorexia.

Syncope: This suggests a more significant bleed.

Drug History: Specifically, aspirin, NSAIDs, warfarin, and iron supplements.

Alcohol Consumption: Could indicate cirrhosis or varices.

Examination

1. Airway, Breathing, Circulation (ABC): Check the basic vital signs and assess for signs of hypovolemic shock (elevated pulse, low BP, altered GCS, cool extremities, prolonged capillary refill).

2. Vomitus and Faeces: Examine any vomit or stools for blood.

3. Abdominal Examination: Look for masses, tenderness, or surgical scars (e.g., from aortic grafts).

4. Signs of Liver Disease: Check for jaundice, spider naevi, or palmar erythema.

5. PR Examination: Check for occult blood in the stool.

Investigation and Diagnosis

Obtain old hospital notes if available.

Order blood tests: FBC, clotting screen, U&E (urea and electrolytes), blood glucose, and Group and Save or cross-matching.

Urea may be elevated, while creatinine typically remains normal unless renal function is impaired.

Check SpO2 (oxygen saturation). Consider an ABG (arterial blood gas) if SpO2 is less than 94%.

CXR (Chest X-ray) and ECG may be necessary based on the patient's condition.

Endoscopy is the primary diagnostic tool to identify the bleeding source.

Risk of Further Bleeding and Mortality

The risk of complications and death increases with:

Age (older patients are at higher risk).

Comorbidities, especially cancer, heart failure, and liver disease.

Ongoing bleeding, elevated urea levels, and PR bleeding.

Initial Rockall Score for Mortality Risk in Upper GI Bleeding

Score	0	1	2	3
Age	<60	60 - 79	>80	
Shock	HR <100, BP <100 mm Hg	BP <100 mm Hg		
Comorbidity	No major comorbidity	Cardiac failure, Ischemic heart disease	Liver failure, renal failure, malignancy	

A score of 0 suggests low risk, and patients may be discharged with follow-up. A score > 0 requires urgent endoscopy.

Treatment of Moderate/Severe Hemorrhage

1. Airway and Breathing: Ensure oxygenation and maintain SpO2 between 94-98%.

2. IV Access: Insert two large-bore (14G) IV cannula.

3. Blood and Fluid Resuscitation: Administer fluids and blood products as needed.

4. Proton Pump Inhibitors: Avoid omeprazole acutely unless the patient has a known peptic ulcer.

5. Anticoagulation Management: If anticoagulated, consult a hematologist and administer Vitamin K, clotting factors, or fresh frozen plasma.

6. Urinary Catheter: Insert a urinary catheter and monitor urine output.

7. Airway Management: In cases of severe bleeding or varices, secure the airway (consider intubation).

Managing Severe Hemorrhage from Varices

For patients with variceal bleeding (commonly in those with cirrhosis or hepatic failure):

1. Fluid Resuscitation: Start IV fluids and administer terlipressin (2 mg IV every 4–6 hours).

2. Coagulation Monitoring: Check INR and administer Vitamin K if prolonged.

3. Prophylactic Antibiotics: Administer ciprofloxacin or a third-generation cephalosporin.

4. Balloon Tamponade: Consider Sengstaken-Minnesota tube for massive hemorrhage. Inflate gastric and esophageal balloons to tamponade the bleeding varices.

Lower Gastrointestinal Bleeding (LGIB)

While the majority of gastrointestinal bleeding originates from the upper GI tract, approximately 20% of cases are due to lower GI causes, including:

Angiodysplasia: Common cause of lower GI bleeding.

Diverticulosis: Another frequent source.

Inflammatory Bowel Disease (IBD) or Aorto-enteric Fistulae (rare).

History

Nature of Bleeding:

Melaena may result from bleeding in the small bowel or proximal colon.

Fresh rectal bleeding could indicate lower GI issues.

Associated Symptoms: Symptoms like weight loss, anorexia, or changes in bowel habits may suggest colonic carcinoma.

Past History: Inquire about IBD, peptic ulcers, or prior aortic surgery (which may cause aorto-enteric fistula).

Medication History: Check for use of NSAIDs, salicylates, or anticoagulants.

Examination

Assess for hypovolemia: Measure pulse, BP, and temperature. Look for any postural drop in BP, indicative of volume loss.

Perform abdominal and PR examination to identify any masses or blood.

Investigation

Obtain blood for cross-matching and FBC, U&E, and coagulation studies.

For older patients, ECG may be required.

Consider imaging studies or endoscopy for definitive localization.

Treatment

1. Resuscitation: Provide oxygen, IV fluids, and monitor vital signs.

2. IV Access: Insert two large-bore cannula.

3. Coagulopathy: Correct any coagulation abnormalities.

4. Consultation: Contact surgical teams for severe cases.

Headache

Headaches are a frequent emergency department (ED) complaint, and while most are benign, a significant portion may signal serious underlying pathology.

Causes of Headache

Primary Headaches:

Migraine

Tension Headaches

Cluster Headaches

Other benign types (e.g., exertional, cough-related).

Secondary Headaches:

Head Injury

Vascular Causes: Stroke, intracranial hemorrhage, and others.

Infection: Meningitis, encephalitis.

Metabolic Disorders: Hypoxia, hypercapnia, CO poisoning.

Craniofacial Disorders: Problems related to the sinuses, teeth, or eyes.

History

Sudden onset or worst headache ever may indicate serious conditions like subarachnoid hemorrhage.

Associated symptoms such as fever or focal neurological deficits suggest infections or strokes.

Change in headache patterns in those over 50 years or with a history of cancer or HIV requires urgent attention.

Examination

Check vital signs, including GCS.

Perform a neurological examination, including tests for papilloedema and signs of meningeal irritation.

Management

Order tests like FBC, ESR, CRP, U&E, and blood glucose.

CT/MRI may be required depending on clinical suspicion.

If infection is suspected, initiate IV antibiotics after obtaining blood cultures.

Migraine

Migraines are a common but often misunderstood condition, with patients typically seeking emergency department (ED) care only when their symptoms deviate from their usual pattern. It's important to differentiate migraines from potentially life-threatening conditions. Although the exact cause of migraines is not fully understood, they involve an initial vasoconstriction followed by vasodilation of both intracranial and extracranial blood vessels, which contributes to the characteristic symptoms.

Presentation

Migraine triggers include fatigue, alcohol consumption, menstruation, use of oral contraceptive pills (OCP), hunger, and specific foods like chocolate, cheese, shellfish, and red wine. A third of patients experience a prodrome that lasts between 5 and 30 minutes, which may involve blurred vision, photophobia, scintillating scotoma (blurred or absent vision with zig-zag lines), malaise, anorexia, and vomiting. Some may also experience mild neurological symptoms like hemiparesis, ataxia, or dysphasia. The headache phase usually lasts 4 to 72 hours, presenting as a throbbing, unilateral pain, though it can be generalized. Common symptoms during the headache phase include photophobia, nausea, and phonophobia.

Rare Forms of Migraine

Hemiplegic Migraine: Characterized by profound hemiplegia before the onset of the headache, which resolves quickly but may persist or resolve slowly in some cases.

Basilar Migraine: Involves brain stem symptoms such as vertigo, dysarthria, diplopia, and limb weakness, with impaired consciousness.

Ophthalmoplegic Migraine: Features transient, unilateral ophthalmoplegia and ptosis that may last several days.

Acephalgic Migraine: A rare form where neurological deficits appear without a headache.

Examination

When a patient presents with migraine-like symptoms, it is essential to rule out other serious conditions. This requires a thorough neurological examination and consideration of atypical presentations.

Treatment of Acute Attacks

First-line treatments include simple analgesics like paracetamol (1g PO every 4 hours as needed) or NSAIDs, combined with anti-emetics such as metoclopramide (10 mg PO or IV).

Referral for admission should be considered for patients with neurological signs, altered mental status, or those with uncertain diagnoses, including a change in headache pattern.

If initial treatments are ineffective, more potent medications may be considered, though they come with significant side effects. For example, sumatriptan (6mg SC, 50mg PO, or 20mg intranasally) is effective but should be used cautiously due to its vasoconstrictive properties, which are contraindicated in patients with ischemic heart disease, uncontrolled hypertension, and certain migraine types like basilar and hemiplegic migraines.

Ergotamine is also an option but should generally be avoided due to side effects such as nausea, vomiting, and abdominal pain. It is contraindicated in patients with peripheral vascular disease, ischemic heart disease, pregnancy, breastfeeding, and certain migraine variants.

Other Causes of Headache

1. Cluster Headache

These headaches are more common in men and often have a family history. They typically occur at night, waking the patient, and can be triggered by alcohol. Cluster headaches are characterized by severe, unilateral pain, usually around the eye, and are associated with autonomic symptoms like lacrimation, nasal congestion, and ptosis. Treatment often involves high-flow oxygen therapy (12L/min for 15 minutes), NSAIDs, or paracetamol. Sumatriptan and ergotamine may also be considered under medical guidance.

2. Trigeminal Neuralgia

This condition is characterized by severe, unilateral pain along the distribution of the trigeminal nerve, often triggered by simple stimuli like touch or chewing. Treatment involves carbamazepine and analgesia. Hospitalization may be necessary for severe, unrelieved pain.

3. Tension Headache

Tension headaches are typically continuous, with a pressing or "band-like" sensation. They are often described in dramatic terms by patients and are usually temporal or occipital. There is no associated worsening with exertion, and usual migraine symptoms are absent. Diagnosis is made after excluding other serious causes. Treatment consists of simple analgesics and reassurance.

4. Cranial Arteritis (Giant Cell Arteritis)

This condition should be suspected in patients over 50 with a new-onset headache or change in headache pattern. Associated symptoms may include weight loss, fever, jaw claudication, and visual disturbances (up to 10% may present with acute vision loss). Temporal artery tenderness, thickening, and absent pulses are key examination findings. Immediate treatment with corticosteroids (IV hydrocortisone or oral prednisolone) is crucial to prevent visual loss. Diagnosis is confirmed by temporal artery biopsy.

5. Space-Occupying Lesions
Headaches that persist on the same side or worsen when lying down or straining may indicate space-occupying lesions such as brain tumors or arteriovenous malformations.

6. Malignant Hypertension
Severe headaches may occur in patients with diastolic blood pressure >130mmHg, often due to malignant hypertension.

7. Ventricular Shunts
Headaches associated with a ventricular shunt, particularly if there is drowsiness, should prompt

an urgent referral for suspected infection or blockage.

8. Analgesic Headache

Chronic use of analgesics or medications such as ergotamine, sympathomimetics, and opioids can cause headaches. Withdrawal from substances like caffeine or starting medications like OCP can also be triggers.

9. Cerebral Venous Thrombosis

This condition presents with a sudden-onset headache, nausea, and vomiting, and may be linked to factors like pregnancy or sinus infections. The diagnosis is often missed on CT scans, but an elevated intracranial pressure (ICP) on lumbar puncture can be a clue.

Acute Confusional State (Delirium)

Definition

Delirium is a rapid-onset, fluctuating disturbance in consciousness and cognition, often with perceptual distortions and hallucinations. It can present with a variety of symptoms, including agitation, drowsiness, or stupor, and is commonly worse at night.

Causes of Acute Confusion

Delirium may be triggered by a range of factors, often occurring concurrently:

Medications: Digoxin, steroids, anticholinergics, and diuretics

Substance use: Alcohol, opioids, and hallucinogens

Infections: Pneumonia, UTI, and meningitis

Metabolic disturbances: Hypoxia, hypoglycemia, and electrolyte imbalances

Cardiac events: Acute myocardial infarction (MI) or heart failure

Neurological issues: Head injury or postictal state

Endocrine disorders: Thyroid dysfunction or diabetes

Organ failure: Respiratory, renal, or hepatic failure

Approach

A systematic approach to identify the underlying cause of delirium is essential. This involves a thorough history (if possible, from other sources), physical examination, and baseline investigations.

Investigations for Acute Confusion

A comprehensive examination should include:

Blood tests (e.g., U&E, FBC, blood glucose)

ECG

CXR

Urinalysis

Oxygen saturation and arterial blood gasses (ABG)

Additional tests like blood cultures, serum paracetamol levels, CT scans, and lumbar puncture may be needed depending on clinical suspicion.

Dementia

Dementia involves irreversible cognitive decline and occurs with a preserved level of consciousness. Alzheimer's disease, vascular dementia, and Lewy body dementia are common causes. However, patients with dementia are also at risk of developing delirium from acute illnesses or metabolic changes. An acute worsening of mental status in a patient with dementia should prompt consideration of delirium.

Management of the Unconscious Patient: A Comprehensive Approach

Initial Resuscitation

The unconscious patient requires immediate attention, with priority given to airway, breathing, and circulation. These vital components should be addressed promptly to prevent further complications and ensure the best possible outcomes.

Airway Management:
Regardless of the cause of unconsciousness, airway obstruction or respiratory depression can

lead to fatal consequences or permanent brain damage. Therefore, securing and protecting the airway should be the first step. If trauma is suspected, it is crucial to immobilize the cervical spine immediately.

Breathing:
In cases where the patient shows inadequate breathing, ventilation with oxygen should be initiated using a self-expanding bag with an oxygen reservoir. If the patient appears to be breathing adequately, they should be positioned in the recovery position to reduce the risk of airway obstruction. Vital signs such as the respiratory rate (RR) should be recorded.

Circulation:
Pulse and blood pressure (BP) must be assessed promptly. Additionally, the patient's skin should be evaluated for signs of pallor, cyanosis, sweating, and temperature changes. Establish reliable venous access and monitor the ECG. If necessary, fluid replacement should be administered intravenously.

Level of Consciousness

The Glasgow Coma Scale (GCS) is essential for evaluating the patient's level of consciousness and neurological status. Blood glucose levels should be checked immediately using a blood glucose meter (BGM), and hypoglycemia should be addressed without delay. Pupil size should be recorded for further assessment of neurological function. For patients with a history of alcoholism or suspected malnutrition, slow intravenous thiamine should be administered (e.g., Pabrinex® 2 pairs of ampoules in 100 mL 5% glucose over 30 minutes).

Common Causes of Unconsciousness

Frequent causes include:

Hypoglycemia

Drug overdose

Head injury

Stroke

Subarachnoid hemorrhage

Seizures

Alcohol intoxication

Less common causes encompass:

Type 2 respiratory failure

Cardiac failure and arrhythmias

Hypovolemic shock

Anaphylaxis

Hepatic/renal failure

Hypothermia/hyperthermia

Meningitis/encephalitis

Malaria

Diabetic ketoacidosis (DKA) or hyperosmolar hyperglycemic state (HHS)

Non-convulsive status epilepticus

Wernicke's encephalopathy

Patient History

Obtaining a thorough history is essential. Information should be gathered from both the ambulance crew and family members or friends of the patient. Key questions include:

How was the patient found?

When was the patient last seen conscious?

Are there any signs of trauma?

Is there a history of seizures?

Has the patient traveled abroad recently?

Are there any notable previous symptoms or medical conditions, including depression?

What medications or substances are available?

Checking past medical records, including previous emergency department (ED) notes, may provide crucial insights.

Physical Examination

A comprehensive examination is critical to identify the underlying cause of the patient's condition. Special attention should be paid to the patient's clothing and belongings, which may reveal pertinent information, such as medication containers or medical bracelets indicating pre-existing health conditions.

Respiratory Rate Assessment:
Abnormal respiratory patterns can indicate various conditions. For instance, rapid, irregular breathing may suggest brainstem compression or damage, while slow, labored breathing could be a sign of respiratory depression due to poisoning (e.g., opioids, barbiturates, or tricyclic antidepressants). Respiratory issues might also point to conditions such as aspiration pneumonia, diabetic ketoacidosis, or liver/renal failure.

Pulse and Blood Pressure Monitoring:

Bradycardia: Could be caused by hypoxia, complete heart block, increased intracranial pressure (ICP), or poisoning from digoxin or beta-blockers.

Tachycardia: May indicate hypoxia, hypovolemia, supraventricular tachycardia

(SVT), ventricular tachycardia (VT), or anticholinergic overdose.

Hypotension: Often associated with shock (e.g., hypovolemic, anaphylactic, septic), hypoxia, or poisoning.

Hypertension: Common in patients with increased ICP.

Skin examination should include checking for pallor, cyanosis, jaundice, rashes (e.g., meningococcal infection), or signs of trauma (e.g., injection marks in cases of drug use). Any evidence of prolonged unconsciousness, such as erythema or blistering over pressure points, is significant.

Neurological Examination

Neurological examination should assess consciousness using GCS, limb strength, reflexes, pupil size, and neck stiffness (if trauma is not suspected). The presence of lateralizing signs such as facial or limb weakness may indicate a stroke, intracranial hemorrhage, or pre-existing neurological conditions (e.g., previous stroke or Bell's palsy).

Wernicke's encephalopathy may manifest as ocular nerve palsy or divergent squint, requiring thiamine administration.

Seizure activity can sometimes be subtle, appearing as eyelid or ocular muscle twitching. These signs should raise suspicion for non-convulsive status epilepticus.

Subhyaloid hemorrhages (blotchy hemorrhages in the retina) are indicative of subarachnoid hemorrhage.

Hypoglycemia may mimic stroke symptoms, presenting with localized weakness or coma. Coma without lateralizing signs is commonly caused by poisoning, postictal states, brainstem strokes, or hepatic failure. Extensor plantar reflexes often appear in such cases.

Diagnostic Investigations

Key investigations to help diagnose the cause of unconsciousness include:

Blood glucose levels: If hypoglycemia is suspected, treatment should be started immediately, even before laboratory results are confirmed.

Arterial blood gasses (ABG): Necessary for evaluating the patient's oxygenation status and overall acid-base balance.

Full blood count (FBC), prothrombin time, and urea and electrolytes (U&E): To assess for underlying causes such as infections, bleeding disorders, or electrolyte imbalances.

Drug levels: Check for paracetamol, salicylates, and other drugs if poisoning is suspected.

ECG: To identify arrhythmias or other cardiovascular abnormalities.

Chest X-ray (CXR): Useful for identifying conditions like pneumonia, aspiration, trauma, or tumors.

CT scan: Essential for detecting intracranial hemorrhage, stroke, or head injuries.

Psychogenic Coma

In rare cases, patients may present with psychogenic coma, in which unconsciousness is feigned. This can be difficult to diagnose definitively. It should be considered only after other causes have been ruled out. One clue is the presence of Bell's phenomenon, where the eyes deviate upwards, showing only the sclera when the eyes are opened.

Collapse and Syncope

Syncope is characterized by a sudden, brief loss of consciousness, followed by spontaneous recovery.

Key Considerations:

Identify life-threatening causes and initiate treatment immediately.

Determine the need for admission or follow-up care for the patient.

Evaluating a Syncope Episode

Is it simply fainting? Vasovagal syncope is often triggered by environmental factors such as heat, prolonged standing, sudden fright, or visual stimuli (e.g., blood). Other causes may include large meals, dehydration, or alcohol consumption. Typically, this is preceded by symptoms like dizziness, nausea, tiredness, yawning, blurred vision, or altered hearing. In some cases, if the individual cannot lie down, seizure-like movements (convulsive syncope) may occur, and there could be vomiting or incontinence, which are not reliable indicators of a seizure.

Is it a seizure? Review emergency records and obtain witness accounts. Seizures often lack prodromal symptoms but may be preceded by a cry, followed by tonic-clonic movements. Cyanosis, frothing at the mouth, heavy breathing, tongue biting, and incontinence suggest a generalized seizure. Post-ictal confusion or drowsiness is normal; however, a very rapid recovery casts doubt on the diagnosis of a seizure.

Could it be a cardiac event? Cardiac syncope typically presents suddenly (e.g., due to hypertrophic cardiomyopathy) and is often accompanied by pallor and sweating. Recovery can be rapid, with some patients experiencing flushing or sighing respirations (e.g., in

Stokes-Adams attacks). Nausea and vomiting are not typically associated with cardiac-related syncope. Inquire about previous episodes, chest pain, palpitations, and any family history of sudden death. Syncope during exertion may indicate aortic or mitral stenosis, pulmonary hypertension, cardiomyopathy, or coronary artery disease.

Other causes: Carotid sinus syncope occurs when the carotid sinus is overstimulated, often during shaving or head-turning. Medications (e.g., GTN, beta-blockers) can also induce syncope. Rare but serious causes include subarachnoid hemorrhage, ruptured ectopic pregnancy, aortic or carotid dissection, pulmonary embolism (PE), or gastrointestinal bleeding. Transient ischemic attack (TIA) is a rare cause of syncope.

Assessment and Management:

Upon a patient's sudden loss of consciousness in the ED:

Assess responsiveness and pulse.

Ensure airway patency, administer oxygen, and monitor pulse and ECG.

Record neurological signs, measure blood pressure (BP), and oxygen saturation (SpO2).

For patients presenting after syncope:

Obtain a detailed history from both the patient and witnesses.

Examine the cardiovascular system for murmurs, arrhythmias, or abnormalities.

Perform a neurological exam to check for focal deficits.

Conduct postural tests (supine and standing pulse/BP measurements). Postural hypotension is common, but significant symptoms like dizziness or weakness should prompt further investigation for causes such as hypovolemia (e.g., GI bleed or ectopic pregnancy).

Perform tests such as blood glucose measurement to rule out hypoglycemia and an ECG to detect arrhythmias, left ventricular hypertrophy (LVH), ischemia, or prior or acute myocardial infarction (MI). An abnormal ECG may reveal conditions such as hypertrophic cardiomyopathy (HCM) or Brugada syndrome.

Disposition:

Admit patients for cardiology evaluation if they have:

Abnormal ECG findings.

Heart failure.

Loss of consciousness with exertion.

Family history of sudden death before age 40 or inherited cardiac conditions.

Age over 65 years with no prodromal symptoms.

A heart murmur.

Refer patients to an epilepsy specialist if they present with:

Tongue biting.

Amnesia, unusual posturing, or prolonged limb jerking.

A history of prodromal symptoms.

Post-ictal confusion.

Patients who fully recover, show signs of vasovagal syncope, and have normal exams may be safely discharged.

Diagnoses Not to Miss:

Gastrointestinal (GI) bleed: Syncope with postural symptoms may suggest significant blood loss and hypovolemia. A rectal exam should be performed to check for blood or melena.

Ectopic pregnancy: Women with syncope and abdominal pain or gynecological symptoms should undergo a pregnancy test.

Ruptured abdominal aortic aneurysm (AAA).

Pulmonary embolism (PE): A witness may report cyanosis, which may indicate a large thrombus.

Acute Generalized Weakness

Generalized weakness can be a symptom of common neurological conditions (e.g., TIA or stroke) or can occur in cases of collapse (refer to Collapse and Syncope section). Less frequently, it is seen in various diseases.

Possible Causes:

Guillain-Barré Syndrome: Following a viral respiratory or GI infection, this syndrome is characterized by progressive, symmetrical weakness that begins distally and moves proximally. Symptoms include muscle tenderness, back pain, loss of reflexes, sensory disturbances (e.g., paraesthesias), and autonomic dysfunction (e.g., hypertension, tachycardia, bladder atony). Be vigilant for respiratory failure, which can progress to respiratory arrest. Serial vital capacity measurements should be taken. ICU referral may be required.

Multiple Sclerosis (MS): This demyelinating CNS disease typically affects women aged

20-50. It presents with relapsing-remitting symptoms such as leg weakness, ataxia, sensory loss, autonomic dysfunction (e.g., bladder issues), and diplopia. Patients may also present with optic neuritis, which causes pain and visual blurring in one eye. Refer to neurology for further management, and if eye symptoms are present, urgent ophthalmology consultation may be required.

Polymyositis: This inflammatory myopathy presents with symmetrical proximal muscle weakness and arthritis, sometimes with muscle tenderness. Patients may have difficulty performing tasks like climbing stairs or brushing hair. Elevated creatine kinase (CK) levels are common. Referral to a rheumatologist is recommended.

Myasthenia Gravis: This rare autoimmune disorder results in fatigable muscle weakness, particularly in the cranial muscles (e.g., ptosis, diplopia). Tendon reflexes and pupil responses are typically unaffected. Myasthenic crisis, marked by severe muscle weakness, may require temporary ventilatory support. New or under-treated cases require referral for diagnostic testing, including the edrophonium test.

Periodic Paralysis: A family of inherited conditions affecting muscle ion channels, episodes of weakness are often associated with fluctuations in serum potassium. Hypokalemic periodic paralysis responds to oral potassium supplementation.

Wound Botulism: Botulism has resurged in the IV drug-using population. It results from infection with Clostridium botulinum, which inhibits acetylcholine release, causing symptoms like diplopia, ptosis, and neck weakness, potentially leading to respiratory failure. Treatment involves antitoxin, antibiotics (penicillin and metronidazole), and respiratory support.

Other Causes of Generalized Weakness:

Spinal cord compression

Tetanus

Alcoholic myopathy

Diphtheria

Lead poisoning

Stroke

A stroke is defined as an acute neurological deficit of vascular origin, lasting for more than 24 hours. The brain's blood supply comes from two primary sources: the internal carotid arteries and the basilar artery. The internal carotids supply the anterior and middle cerebral arteries, forming the anterior circulation, while the basilar artery supplies the posterior cerebral arteries, known as the posterior circulation. The circle of

Willis, through anterior and posterior communicating arteries, provides collateral circulation in cases of carotid artery stenosis.

Pathogenesis

Approximately 70% of strokes occur in individuals over 70 years of age, though strokes can affect people of any age. The two main types of stroke are:

1. Cerebral Infarction (80%):

Thrombosis caused by atherosclerosis, hypertension, and occasionally arteritis.

Cerebral Embolism from conditions such as atrial fibrillation (AF), valvular heart disease, myocardial infarction (MI), ventricular aneurysm, myxoma, endocarditis, or cardiomyopathy.

Hypoperfusion episodes leading to reduced blood supply.

2. Cerebral Hemorrhage (20%):

Primarily associated with hypertension, which can lead to the rupture of small arteries in the brain.

Subarachnoid hemorrhage.

Conditions like bleeding disorders (e.g., anticoagulant use) and intracranial tumors.

Presentation

A stroke may be preceded by neck pain, indicating carotid or vertebral artery dissection or subarachnoid hemorrhage.

Headache, while uncommon in strokes, may indicate a cerebral hemorrhage.

A differential diagnosis is essential to rule out other potential conditions (e.g., hypoglycemia, Todd's paresis, hemiplegic migraine, meningitis, encephalitis, brain abscess, head injury, Bell's palsy, and 'Saturday night palsy').

A thorough examination should include:

Mental status assessment (Glasgow Coma Scale) and signs of meningeal irritation.

Head and neck injury examination.

Pupil, fundus, and cranial nerve examination.

Motor function assessment (tone, power, reflexes).

Sensory function examination, including speech and comprehension.

Cerebellar signs (coordination, speech).

Sources of embolism (e.g., AF, murmurs, carotid bruits).

Accurate localization based solely on clinical grounds can be challenging, and the differentiation between infarction and hemorrhage requires CT/MRI imaging. The ROSIER score can be used to identify patients with acute stroke, although it may miss posterior circulation infarcts.

Investigation

Initial investigations should exclude other potential causes and confirm the diagnosis of stroke. Basic investigations include:

BMG, FBC, ESR, U&E, blood glucose, ECG, and CXR. Continuous monitoring with pulse oximetry (ABG if SpO2 <94%) and cardiac monitoring is essential.

Emergency CT

Patients presenting with symptoms within 4 hours of onset, potentially eligible for thrombolysis treatment.

Patients on anticoagulants or with a known bleeding disorder.

Glasgow Coma Scale (GCS) <13 or unexplained fluctuating symptoms.

Papilloedema, neck stiffness, fever, or a severe headache at symptom onset.

Management

Hypoglycemia should be corrected immediately if present.

Blood pressure (BP) is often elevated early after a stroke; however, avoid attempting to lower BP at presentation unless necessary.

Oxygen supplementation is advised if SpO2 <95%.

Swallowing assessment should be performed (e.g., offering a teaspoon of water).

If intracranial hemorrhage is excluded, administer aspirin 300mg orally or rectally if the patient is unable to swallow. If allergic to aspirin, use an alternative antiplatelet such as clopidogrel.

Whenever possible, patients should be admitted to specialized stroke units for treatment and rehabilitation.

Thrombolysis

If intracranial hemorrhage is excluded within 4 hours of symptom onset, alteplase may be administered in an appropriate acute stroke service setting. Local guidelines and NICE recommendations should be followed.

Transient Ischemic Attacks (TIA)

A TIA is a brief episode of focal neurological deficit of vascular origin, lasting less than 24 hours. TIAs serve as a significant warning for future stroke risk, with up to 5% of patients experiencing a stroke within 48 hours and up to 50% within 5 years. Even if symptoms resolve, most patients show evidence of infarction on CT/MRI.

Presentation

Carotid territory involvement leads to unilateral weakness, sensory changes, dysphasia, homonymous hemianopia, or amaurosis .

Vertebrobasilar territory involvement causes blackouts, bilateral motor or sensory changes, vertigo, and ataxia.

Causes

Most TIAs are caused by thrombo-embolic disease, from:

Cardiac sources: AF, mitral stenosis, artificial heart valves, post-MI.

Extracranial sources: Carotid artery stenosis. Other causes include:

Hypertension

Polycythaemia/anemia

Vasculitis (temporal arteritis, SLE)

Sickle cell disease

Hypoglycemia

Hypoperfusion (e.g., arrhythmia, hypovolemia)

Syphilis

Assessment

To diagnose a TIA, symptoms must resolve within 24 hours. A thorough neurological examination and documentation of vital signs are essential. Investigations should focus on identifying potential embolic sources (e.g., AF, heart murmurs, carotid bruits, MI).

Investigations

BMG, FBC, ESR, U&E, blood glucose, lipids, and INR (if on anticoagulants).

ECG to assess for MI, arrhythmias.

Additional imaging (e.g., carotid Doppler, MRI).

Management

Calculate the ABCD2 score to assess the risk of stroke after a TIA.

Admit patients with a score of 4 or more or those with multiple TIAs in the previous week to a stroke unit.

Aspirin (300mg) should be started immediately.

For patients with continuing symptoms or deficits, admission is warranted.

Seizures and Status Epilepticus

First Seizure

A detailed history is essential for diagnosing a first seizure. Witnessed events should be documented clearly, distinguishing them from other causes of collapse, such as syncope. Conditions such as hypoglycemia, stroke, infections (e.g., meningitis), and metabolic disturbances should be considered.

Status Epilepticus

Status epilepticus is characterized by continuous generalized seizures lasting more than 30 minutes or recurrent seizures without intervening recovery. It can result from cerebral infections, trauma, cerebrovascular disease, and metabolic disturbances.

Management of Status Epilepticus

1. Airway management: Clear the airway and provide high-flow oxygen.

2. Seizure control: Administer IV lorazepam (4mg) and repeat if necessary.

3. Correct hypoglycemia: Administer IV glucose (20% solution).

4. Investigate underlying causes: Check for infections, metabolic disturbances, and other contributing factors.

Note: Further treatment, including antiepileptic drugs and possibly magnesium sulfate (for eclampsia), may be required depending on the underlying cause. Always consider potential complications such as hypoxia and increased intracranial pressure (ICP).

Sodium Imbalance and Management:

Abnormal sodium levels can arise in conditions such as hypervolaemia, euvolaemia, or hypovolaemia, each associated with different pathophysiological causes. The management of these conditions must be tailored to the underlying imbalance.

Hypernatraemia: Hypernatraemia can result from several causes, including diabetes insipidus (either due to insufficient ADH or renal resistance to ADH), diarrhea, vomiting, the use of diuretics, hypertonic saline, sodium bicarbonate, or Cushing's syndrome. In treating hypernatraemia, sodium levels should be corrected slowly, not exceeding a 1 mmol/L/hour increase. For patients with hypovolaemia (manifesting as tachycardia, hypotension, or postural hypotension), initial treatment includes 0.9% saline. Once the patient reaches a normal fluid status (euvolaemia), a more dilute solution like 0.45% saline or 5% dextrose should be used. The free water deficit can be calculated using the formula:

Free water deficit (liters) = $0.6 \times$ weight (kg) $\times$ (serum Na / 140 - 1), with replacement typically over a 48-hour period. This should be in addition to regular maintenance fluids. Serum sodium should be monitored 2–3 hours after treatment to ensure a safe and gradual correction.

Potential complications of hypernatraemia include seizures, subdural and intracerebral hemorrhages, ischemic stroke, and dural sinus thrombosis. Rapid correction, particularly in cases of chronic hypernatraemia, can cause cerebral edema and exacerbate neurological issues.

Hyponatraemia: The causes of hyponatraemia are varied, including excessive fluid loss replaced with hypotonic fluids (e.g., diarrhea, burns, prolonged exercise), polydipsia, ecstasy ingestion, syndrome of inappropriate ADH secretion, nephrotic syndrome, renal dysfunction, liver cirrhosis, cardiac failure, and various medications such as diuretics and ACE inhibitors.

Acute Hyponatremia (<24 hours): For patients with mild symptoms, fluid restriction may be sufficient. However, those presenting with seizures or signs of raised intracranial pressure (ICP) are at a higher risk and require more aggressive management. A serum sodium level below 120 mmol/L is associated with a high risk of brain herniation. In these cases, up to 200mL of 2.7% saline can be administered intravenously over 30 minutes, with re-evaluation of serum sodium levels afterward.

Chronic Hyponatremia (>24 hours): Correcting chronic hyponatremia should be done cautiously to avoid central pontine myelinolysis, especially in patients with low potassium levels or those who are alcohol-dependent. Sodium should be corrected no faster than 10 mmol/L per 24 hours. Treatment involves addressing the underlying cause (e.g., discontinuing diuretics). Fluid restriction is necessary for hypovolemic patients, such as those with heart failure, cirrhosis, or nephrotic syndrome. Severe cases of hyponatremia with seizures or altered mental status may be treated with hypertonic saline (200mL of 2.7% saline over 30 minutes), aiming to raise the serum sodium by no more than 5 mmol/L.

Addisonian Crisis: An Addisonian crisis refers to acute adrenal insufficiency, which is often precipitated by the sudden cessation of chronic steroid therapy or by stressors such as infections or trauma. The most common cause of Addison's disease is autoimmune (idiopathic), accounting for about 80% of cases in the UK. It is associated with other autoimmune disorders like Graves' disease, Hashimoto's thyroiditis, type 1 diabetes, and others.

Precipitating Factors:

Infection, trauma, myocardial infarction (MI), cerebral infarction, asthma, alcohol use, pregnancy, or reduction in steroid therapy.

Clinical Presentation: Addison's disease often presents insidiously with nonspecific symptoms such as weakness, fatigue, anorexia, weight loss, and abdominal pain. During a crisis, patients may experience shock (tachycardia, peripheral vasoconstriction, severe hypotension, syncope), oliguria, muscle weakness, confusion, and hypoglycaemia. Chronic features include hyperpigmentation and vitiligo.

Investigations: Lab findings may include hyperkalemia, hyponatraemia, hypoglycaemia, mild acidosis, and eosinophilia. If Addisonian crisis is suspected, treatment should begin immediately, even before lab results are available.

Management:

Secure intravenous access.

Draw blood for cortisol and ACTH levels.

Administer hydrocortisone sodium succinate (100mg IV).

If the patient is hypotensive, begin volume resuscitation with 0.9% saline.

Correct hypoglycemia with 50mL of 10% glucose IV.

Consider broad-spectrum antibiotics if infection is suspected.

Urgent referral for hospitalization is necessary.

Thyrotoxic Crisis (Thyroid Storm): Thyrotoxic crisis is a rare but severe condition that can occur in patients with hyperthyroidism, particularly those with Graves' disease. Mortality can be high (8–10%).

Causes: This condition is often triggered by a stressor such as:

Premature cessation of anti-thyroid treatment.

Recent surgery or radio-iodine therapy.

Infections (especially chest infections).

Trauma, diabetic ketoacidosis (DKA), thyroid hormone overdose, and pre-eclampsia.

Clinical Features: Symptoms include fever, tachycardia, agitation, confusion, abdominal pain, diarrhea, and sometimes arrhythmias. It may mimic an acute abdomen or sepsis.

Differential Diagnosis: Conditions that may resemble thyrotoxic crisis include neuroleptic malignant syndrome, septic shock, or anticholinergic overdose.

Investigations:

U&E, BMG, and blood glucose levels.

TSH, T3, and T4 levels.

ECG to assess for arrhythmias.

CXR to look for signs of infection or heart failure.

Management:

Secure the airway and provide oxygen if needed.

Administer intravenous fluids (0.9% saline).

Consider a nasogastric tube if vomiting persists.

Sedate with benzodiazepines (e.g., diazepam) or haloperidol.

Give dexamethasone or hydrocortisone to manage thyroid hormone levels.

Start broad-spectrum antibiotics if an infection is suspected.

Cooling measures may be required for hyperthermia.

Once stabilized, treatment with beta-blockers (e.g., propranolol), carbimazole, and iodine is initiated. Aspirin should be avoided as it can displace thyroid hormones from binding proteins.

Urinary Tract Infection (UTI): A UTI occurs when bacteria invade the urinary tract, and the presence of $\geq 10^5$ colony-forming units per mL of urine indicates infection. UTIs are more common in females due to a shorter urethra, and E. coli is the most common pathogen.

Presentation:

Lower UTI (Cystitis): Symptoms include dysuria, frequency, urgency, and suprapubic discomfort.

Upper UTI (Pyelonephritis): This presents with fever, loin pain, vomiting, and malaise, and can lead to sepsis in severe cases.

Investigation: Urinalysis (dipstick) may show signs of infection such as haematuria, leucocytes, and nitrites. A urine culture (MSU) is essential to identify the specific pathogen and guide antibiotic treatment.

Treatment:

For uncomplicated lower UTIs in women, a 3–6 day course of trimethoprim or nitrofurantoin is typically effective.

For pregnant women, both symptomatic and asymptomatic bacteriuria should be treated with antibiotics like amoxicillin.

Elderly patients with asymptomatic bacteriuria typically do not require antibiotics unless they are symptomatic.

Men with suspected prostatitis may require more tailored treatment, and all cases of UTI should involve appropriate follow-up.

Porphyria

Porphyrias are a group of disorders resulting from defects in heme biosynthesis, leading to the accumulation of porphyrins and their precursors. These conditions are mostly hereditary, though they can also arise from factors like iron deficiency, excessive alcohol consumption, and lead poisoning. The acute forms of porphyria (such as acute intermittent porphyria, variegate porphyria, and hereditary coproporphyria) are relatively rare, affecting about 81 in 10,000 people in the UK. On the other hand, non-acute forms (such as porphyria) primarily result in skin sensitivity to light and may be linked with liver disease.

Acute attacks of porphyria can be triggered by certain medications like barbiturates, oral contraceptives, sulfonamides, and others, as well as factors such as alcohol, smoking, emotional or physical stress, infections, and pregnancy.

Clinical Features of Acute Porphyria:

Abdominal pain: Severe, often associated with nausea, vomiting, and constipation. Abdominal examination may show mild tenderness or appear normal.

Peripheral neuropathy: Typically motor, progressing to paralysis and possibly respiratory failure.

Autonomic dysfunction: Tachycardia, hypertension, and postural hypotension are common.

Psychiatric symptoms: These may include agitation, depression, mania, and hallucinations.

Hyponatremia: Caused by inappropriate ADH secretion, which can lead to seizures or coma.

Investigation and Management:

Diagnosis: Look for a Medic-Alert bracelet or previous medical records. If an acute attack is suspected, send a fresh urine sample, protected from light, to test for elevated levels of aminolevulinic acid and porphobilinogen. The urine typically turns dark red or brown when exposed to light.

Supportive Care: Carbohydrate intake (either orally or intravenously) is crucial. Mild pain can be managed with paracetamol or aspirin; more severe pain may require morphine, potentially with an antiemetic. For agitation, consider chlorpromazine, and for severe hypertension, propranolol may be used.

Seizures: Management of status epilepticus in these patients can be challenging, as many anticonvulsants are contraindicated. Diazepam IV is generally preferred.

Specialized treatment: Hem may be helpful for some patients experiencing acute crises, but this requires specialist guidance.

Drug Considerations:

Many drugs can precipitate porphyria attacks, so careful consideration is needed before prescribing. The safety of numerous drugs remains uncertain, and patient responses may vary. For drugs known to be safer, examples include ibuprofen, penicillin, ciprofloxacin, and bupivacaine. Always check with the patient and consult the British National Formulary (BNF) or a specialist when in doubt.

Bleeding Disorders

Hemostasis involves a coordinated process between the vascular system, platelets, and the coagulation cascade to limit blood loss. A primary platelet plug forms through interactions with the vascular subendothelium, reinforced by cross-linked fibrin strands formed via the coagulation cascade, ensuring the integrity of the vessel wall. Excessive clot formation is regulated by the fibrinolytic system, which breaks down fibrin to prevent inappropriate thrombosis.

Recognizing Bleeding Disorders:

Bleeding is expected after trauma, but spontaneous or excessive bleeding without injury, or delayed bleeding (over several hours or days), may suggest a bleeding disorder. These disorders can be congenital or acquired, and the patient's medical history, including any history of abnormal bleeding after dental work, surgery, or trauma, should be reviewed.

Congenital disorders: Common examples include Hemophilia A (Factor VIII deficiency), Hemophilia B (Factor IX deficiency), and von Willebrand's disease. These conditions are often well-known to patients, who typically carry a Medic-Alert bracelet or National Hemophilia card for identification.

Acquired disorders: These may arise due to liver disease, kidney failure, medications (such as aspirin, NSAIDs, warfarin, or alcohol), or underlying conditions like hematologic malignancies. Hypothermia can also exacerbate bleeding tendencies.

Clinical Presentation:

Platelet disorders: These often present with mucocutaneous bleeding (e.g., nosebleeds, heavy menstrual bleeding, bruising). Thrombocytopenia is a common cause, but platelet function may be impaired even with normal platelet counts, such as in the presence of certain drugs like aspirin.

Coagulation disorders: Bleeding into deep tissues or joints, delayed bleeding after trauma or surgery, and the presence of large hematomas are often signs of coagulation factor deficiencies.

Investigations:

Complete Blood Count (CBC): In acute bleeds, hemoglobin and hematocrit values may not accurately reflect blood loss due to hemodilution. A platelet count of less than $100 \times 10^9/L$ indicates thrombocytopenia, and counts under $20 \times 10^9/L$ are associated with spontaneous bleeding.

Prothrombin Time (PT) and INR: These are used to monitor anticoagulant therapy and assess liver function.

Activated Partial Thromboplastin Time (aPTT): This tests the intrinsic and common coagulation pathways.

Factor assays: Specific tests can identify individual clotting factor deficiencies and the presence of inhibitors that may prolong clotting.

General Management of Bleeding Disorders:

Wound care and fracture management: Patients with bleeding disorders require careful management, which may include the administration of clotting factor concentrates or platelets under the guidance of a hematologist.

Intracranial hemorrhage: Always consider the possibility of brain bleeds in patients presenting with neurological symptoms or minor head trauma. Immediate treatment may be required before imaging results are available.

Avoid certain procedures: Intramuscular injections and central line placements are contraindicated due to the risk of uncontrollable bleeding.

Drug interactions: Before prescribing any medication, it is essential to verify whether it may exacerbate the bleeding disorder or interfere with treatment.

Specific Conditions:

Vascular Lesions: These can be inherited (e.g., Ehlers-Danlos syndrome, osteogenesis imperfecta) or acquired due to conditions like vasculitis or scurvy.

Platelet Disorders: Disorders like idiopathic thrombocytopenic purpura (ITP) or disseminated intravascular coagulation (DIC) often present with mucocutaneous bleeding, while deep tissue bleeding is more common in coagulation disorders.

Hemophilia A and B: These genetic disorders result in the deficiency of clotting factors, leading to delayed bleeding, particularly in deep tissues or joints. Treatment typically involves factor replacement therapy.

Disseminated Intravascular Coagulation (DIC):

DIC can occur due to a variety of triggers, including infections, trauma, malignancy, pregnancy complications, or severe shock. It leads to the consumption of clotting factors and platelets, resulting in systemic fibrin deposition and an increased risk of bleeding.

Investigations and Treatment of DIC:

Lab findings: Patients with DIC will often show low platelet counts, prolonged PT and aPTT, decreased fibrinogen, and elevated fibrin degradation products.

Management: The primary approach is to treat the underlying cause. In some cases, expert advice on blood products (platelets, FFP, prothrombin complex) or heparin therapy may be necessary.

Anticoagulant Therapy

Warfarin is a commonly used oral anticoagulant that inhibits the production of vitamin K-dependent clotting factors. Management of patients on warfarin requires regular monitoring of INR levels. If a bleeding event occurs, treatment may include reversal with vitamin K or fresh frozen plasma, depending on the severity of the bleeding.

Blood Transfusion: A Comprehensive Overview

Introduction: Prevention of Blood Loss vs. Transfusion It is preferable to prevent excessive blood loss rather than relying on transfusion to replace it. Proper management of blood transfusion starts with meticulous documentation and labeling, which are critical for patient safety. Accurate identification of the patient and verification of their details are essential before any transfusion. In cases where a patient's details are uncertain, a unique identifier (such as an Emergency Department number) should be used, and the blood transfusion laboratory should be notified.

Labeling and Blood Collection Procedures

Blood samples must be taken by the clinician at the patient's bedside, with immediate labeling of blood tubes to reduce the risk of misidentification. Mislabelled tubes can result in refusal by blood banks to process them. The doctor responsible for collecting the sample should also complete the necessary forms and contact the transfusion service. Only one patient's blood should be drawn at a time to avoid errors.

Additionally, healthcare providers must be vigilant about patients' religious or personal preferences regarding blood products. For example, administering blood to a patient who refuses it on religious grounds (e.g., Jehovah's Witnesses) could lead to serious legal consequences.

Blood Collection Requirements

Typically, 10 mL of clotted blood is sufficient for most adults. In cases where a massive transfusion is anticipated, two 10 mL samples should be sent for testing. The request form should specify the amount of blood required and where it should be delivered, along with the date and signature of the requesting doctor.

Blood Product Requests and Assessments The quantity of blood to be kept available depends on the patient's clinical condition and potential future blood loss. Assessing a patient's blood volume loss, especially in cases of hypovolemic shock, is complex. This includes evaluating clinical signs, estimating blood loss, and conducting relevant investigations. Hemoglobin (Hb) and hematocrit (Hct) levels may not accurately reflect acute blood loss, as it can take hours for these values to stabilize.

Group and Screen: This test determines the patient's ABO and RhD blood group and checks for any unexpected antibodies. If the screen is clear, blood can be provided quickly (within 10-15 minutes).

Cross-Match: A full compatibility test may take up to an hour. However, in urgent cases, ABO and RhD compatible blood can typically be available within 15 minutes after performing an "immediate spin crossmatch."

Emergency Transfusion: In cases of massive blood loss, uncross-matched group O Rhesus-negative blood may be issued immediately.

Types of Blood Products In the UK, blood component therapy is commonly used, where separate components such as red blood cells (RBC), platelets, and plasma are administered based on the patient's needs:

Red Blood Cells (Additive Solution): Each unit (300 mL) is from a single donor and has a hematocrit of 0.55–0.65. A transfusion of 4 mL/kg will increase circulating Hb by approximately 8-10 g/dL.

Whole Blood: A unit contains 530 mL, with 470 mL of blood and 63 mL of preservative solution, and has a hematocrit of 0.35–0.45.

Platelet Concentrate: Either pooled or from a single donor via plateletpheresis.

Fresh Frozen Plasma (FFP): Contains clotting factors and fibrinogen.

Cryoprecipitate: Derived from thawed FFP, rich in factor VIII, fibrinogen, and von Willebrand factor.

Prothrombin Complex Concentrate (PCC): Used to reverse the effects of warfarin and contains vitamin K-dependent factors II, VII, IX, and X.

Transfusion Safety Protocols According to UK Blood Safety & Quality Regulations (2005), transfusion procedures require confirmation by two practitioners to ensure all checks are performed accurately. These include verifying patient identification, matching the blood product label with patient details, checking the expiration date, and inspecting the blood component for signs of contamination or damage. The transfusion must be prescribed, and the signed traceability label should be attached to the patient's records.

Transfusions should only be administered using appropriate giving sets with integral filters, and no medications should be added to blood products. Red cell concentrates can be diluted with 0.9% saline, especially for rapid transfusions. Blood warmers are essential for large or rapid transfusions.

Massive Transfusion Protocol Massive transfusion is defined as the loss of 50% or more of circulating blood volume within 3 hours, requiring coordinated interdisciplinary care. Key steps include:

1. Airway Protection & Oxygen: Ensure the airway is clear and administer high-flow oxygen.

2. Get Help: Involve two nurses and a senior doctor for immediate assistance.

3. IV Access: Insert two large-bore cannulas and start intravenous warm saline.

4. Laboratory Tests: Send blood samples (FBC, U&E, LFTs, coagulation, and cross-match) directly to the lab.

5. Notify Hematology: Alert the lab about potential massive transfusion and request ABO group-specific red cells if the patient is peri-arrest.

6. Surgical Intervention: Call for a senior surgeon to control bleeding as quickly as possible.

7. Transfusion Initiation: Start transfusion if the patient remains tachycardia or hypotension despite initial resuscitation.

During massive transfusion, regular monitoring is essential, including frequent blood tests, platelet transfusion if needed (if platelet count drops below 75×10^9/L), and the administration of FFP to replenish clotting factors.

Complications of Massive Transfusion Several complications can arise during massive transfusion, including:

Hypothermia: Rapid infusion of cold blood products may cause significant hypothermia, which should be managed with a blood warmer.

Electrolyte Imbalances: Citrate used as an anticoagulant in blood products can bind calcium, leading to hypocalcemia, which can impair cardiac function. It may also affect magnesium and potassium levels, causing arrhythmias. Routine monitoring of electrolytes and ECG is critical.

Transfusion Reactions Patients should be closely monitored for transfusion reactions, especially during the first 5-10 minutes of the infusion. Signs of a reaction include fever, shortness of breath, chest pain, abdominal pain, or hypotension. Common reactions include allergic responses (itching, hives, bronchospasm) and more serious conditions like mismatched transfusions or bacterial contamination.

Mismatched Transfusion: The most common cause is clerical error, leading to severe haemolysis and circulatory collapse. In cases of suspected transfusion reactions, the transfusion should be stopped immediately, and the patient should be treated for symptoms while investigations are carried out.

Sickle Cell Disease Sickle cell disease is prevalent in populations of African, Mediterranean, Middle Eastern, and Indian descent. The disease is caused by a mutation in the hemoglobin gene, leading to sickling of red blood cells under certain conditions, such as hypoxia or acidosis. Sickle cells are rigid and can obstruct blood vessels, leading to tissue ischemia and further sickling. Management involves supportive care, including blood transfusion, to alleviate symptoms during sickle cell crises.

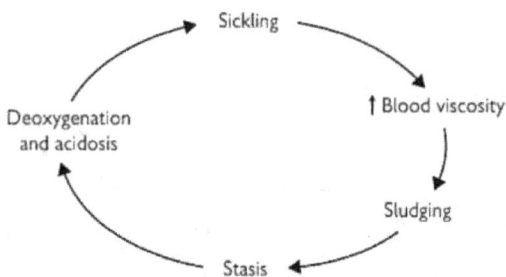

Figure 3-20:Sickling cycle.

Chapter 4
Toxicology

Poisons: General Principles

This section provides foundational knowledge about the nature and classification of poisons, mechanisms of toxicity, and the principles of managing poisoned patients. It highlights the importance of a systematic approach to identifying the toxin and assessing the severity of poisoning.

Diagnosis of Poisoning

Accurate diagnosis is critical in toxicology. This section emphasizes clinical evaluation, patient history, physical examination findings, and the utility of laboratory investigations to confirm exposure and guide management strategies.

Poisons: Supportive Care

Supportive care forms the backbone of poisoning management. Key topics include maintaining airway patency, ensuring adequate breathing and circulation, and monitoring vital signs. The section also covers advanced interventions like mechanical ventilation and hemodynamic support.

Reducing Absorption of Poisons

Discusses methods to limit toxin absorption, including gastric lavage, activated charcoal administration, and whole-bowel irrigation. Evidence-based guidelines on indications, timing, and risks of these interventions are provided.

Antidotes for Poisons

A comprehensive overview of commonly used antidotes, their mechanisms of action, indications, dosing, and contraindications. Case-based examples illustrate the application of antidotes in clinical practice.

Specific Poisonings

Each subsection addresses a specific type of poisoning, detailing clinical features, diagnostic challenges, and evidence-based management protocols:

1. Opioid Poisoning

Symptoms: Respiratory depression, pinpoint pupils, and reduced consciousness.

Management: Administration of naloxone and supportive care.

2. Salicylate Poisoning

Symptoms: Hyperventilation, metabolic acidosis, and tinnitus.

Management: Alkalinization of urine and hemodialysis in severe cases.

3. Paracetamol (Acetaminophen) Poisoning

Symptoms: Asymptomatic phase followed by liver dysfunction.

Management: Early administration of N-acetylcysteine (NAC).

4. Tricyclic Antidepressant Poisoning

Symptoms: Seizures, arrhythmias, and anticholinergic effects.

Management: Sodium bicarbonate for cardiac toxicity.

5. Benzodiazepine Poisoning

Symptoms: CNS depression without significant respiratory compromise.

Management: Flumazenil in specific cases.

6. Barbiturate and Clomethiazole Poisoning

Symptoms: Severe CNS depression.

Management: Supportive care and enhanced elimination techniques.

7. Lithium and Sulfonylurea Poisoning

Lithium: Neurological symptoms; manage with hydration and dialysis.

Sulphonylureas: Hypoglycemia; treat with glucose and octreotide.

8. Beta-Blocker and Calcium Antagonist Poisoning

Symptoms: Bradycardia, hypotension.

Management: High-dose insulin therapy, glucagon, and calcium.

9. Digoxin and ACE Inhibitor Poisoning

Digoxin: Arrhythmias; treat with digoxin-specific antibody fragments.

ACE inhibitors: Manage with supportive care.

10. Iron, Ethanol, Methanol, and Ethylene Glycol Poisoning

Management strategies vary from chelating agents to fomepizole or dialysis.

11. Paraquat, Organophosphates, and Cyanide Poisoning

Paraquat: Minimize absorption; organophosphates: Atropine and pralidoxime; cyanide: Hydroxocobalamin.

12. Carbon Monoxide and Chlorine Poisoning

CO poisoning: Hyperbaric oxygen therapy.

Chlorine poisoning: Supportive care and oxygen supplementation.

Chemical Incidents and Decontamination

Explores response protocols for chemical exposure, including patient decontamination techniques to prevent secondary contamination and environmental spread.

Plants, Berries, Mushrooms, and Button Batteries

Highlights the dangers of accidental ingestion and management principles, including identifying the toxic substance and monitoring for complications.

Illicit Drugs and Serotonin Syndrome

Case-based examples of managing toxicities from illicit drugs like cocaine and amphetamines. Serotonin syndrome management focuses on supportive care and specific therapies like cyproheptadine.

Body Packers

Reviews the risks associated with drug smuggling through internal concealment, diagnostic imaging, and safe retrieval methods.

Principles of Poison Management: A Comprehensive Overview

Emergency Treatment Protocols

1. Airway Management:

Ensure the airway is clear and secure to prevent obstruction.

For patients exhibiting inadequate breathing, administer oxygen via a bag-valve mask or endotracheal (ET) tube. Avoid mouth-to-mouth ventilation, particularly in cases of suspected poisoning.

In opioid-induced respiratory depression, administer naloxone as a specific antidote.

2. Circulatory Support:

Assess the pulse and cardiac status.

Initiate cardiopulmonary resuscitation (CPR) if the patient is unconscious and pulseless.

Categories of Poisoning

1. Unintentional or Accidental Poisoning:

Predominantly seen in children aged 1–4 years, often caused by ingestion of medications, household chemicals, or plants.

Older children and adults may be exposed to toxic chemicals at school, work, or from mishandling household substances.

Medication errors, such as dosing miscalculations or duplicate consumption of drugs with different brand names, are common causes in adults.

2. Deliberate Self-Poisoning:

Most frequent in adults and occasionally in children as young as six years old.

Commonly involves impulsive ingestion of medications or toxins, often driven by emotional distress or to influence others.

All such cases warrant a thorough psychiatric evaluation to assess suicidal intent or underlying psychological issues.

3. Non-Accidental Poisoning in Children:

A rare but severe form of fabricated illness (formerly termed Munchausen's syndrome by proxy) where a caregiver intentionally poisons a child.

4. Homicidal and Terrorism-Related Poisoning:

Involves acute or chronic administration of lethal chemicals like arsenic or thallium.

Chemical plant accidents and bioterrorism pose risks of mass poisoning.

Resources for Poison Identification

1. Drug Identification Tools:

Utilize resources such as the MIMS Colour Index or the British National Formulary (BNF) for tablet identification.

Advanced tools like TIC TAC, a computerized tablet and capsule identification system, provide valuable support.

2. Plant and Fungi Identification:

Identification is challenging but can be aided by specialized reference texts or the interactive software Poisonous Plants and Fungi in Britain and Ireland.

Local botanical experts may also assist in identifying toxic plant species.

3. National Poisons Information Services (UK):

TOXBASE, a clinical toxicology database, is an essential resource for healthcare professionals, offering detailed guidance on managing various types of poisoning.

Clinical Assessment and Monitoring

1. History and Examination:

Gather information from the patient or bystanders about the nature and quantity of the ingested substance.

Evaluate for physical signs of poisoning, such as injection marks, and rule out other conditions like head injuries or meningitis.

2. Toxidrome Recognition:

Opioids: Pinpoint pupils, respiratory depression.

Tricyclic Antidepressants: Coma, dilated pupils, tachycardia.

Salicylates: Tinnitus, hyperventilation, sweating.

3. Vital Signs and Investigations:

Monitor consciousness, respiratory rate, blood glucose, blood pressure, and temperature.

Perform arterial blood gas (ABG) analysis and record electrocardiograms (ECGs) for cardiac monitoring.

Supportive Care Measures

1. Airway Protection:

Use a cuffed ET tube in unconscious patients without a gag reflex. Position the patient to minimize aspiration risks.

2. Managing Hypotension:

Treat with intravenous fluids (e.g., saline). For persistent low blood pressure, consider inotropes like dopamine or dobutamine under specialist guidance.

3. Cardiac Arrhythmias:

Rare but may occur with specific drugs like tricyclic antidepressants or beta-blockers. Focus on correcting underlying causes such as hypoxia or electrolyte imbalances.

4. Seizure Control:

Address prolonged or recurrent seizures with IV lorazepam. Monitor for complications like hypoxia or acidosis.

5. Temperature Dysregulation:

Manage hypothermia with passive rewarming and monitor for hyperthermia in stimulant poisoning cases, providing active cooling and medications as needed.

Reducing Poison Absorption

1. Activated Charcoal:

Administer promptly to bind ingested toxins, provided the patient presents within an appropriate time frame post-ingestion.

2. Gastric Lavage:

Reserved for severe cases under expert guidance to remove toxic substances from the stomach.

Psychiatric and Long-Term Care

1. Post-Poisoning Management:

Patients admitted for observation benefit from a "cooling-off" period to reassess their situation and reduce the likelihood of repeated self-poisoning.

Psychiatric evaluation is crucial for identifying underlying mental health disorders and preventing recurrence.

2. Children's Care:

Admit symptomatic children for monitoring and ensure a safe discharge plan with proper home education to prevent future incidents.

Antidotes and Treatment Protocols for Poisoning

Effective management of poisoning relies on supportive care, with antidotes reserved for specific cases. Below is a simplified guide to commonly used antidotes and their applications, emphasizing professional clarity and accuracy.

For poisoning with metals such as arsenic, lead, mercury, and thallium, chelation therapy is essential. This treatment binds toxic metals to form complexes that are excreted, but it requires specialist consultation to determine appropriate agents and dosages.

In opioid poisoning, common substances include morphine, heroin, and methadone. Symptoms often manifest as coma, pinpoint pupils, respiratory depression, cyanosis, and hypotension. Immediate management involves clearing the airway, providing oxygen, and administering naloxone as the antidote. Naloxone should be initiated at a low dose (e.g., 0.1 mg intravenously) in opioid-dependent individuals to avoid precipitating withdrawal.

Salicylate poisoning, frequently caused by aspirin ingestion, presents with symptoms such as vomiting, tinnitus, hyperventilation, and confusion. Activated charcoal is effective if administered within the first hour of ingestion. Gastric lavage may be considered in cases where the ingested dose exceeds 500 mg/kg. Monitoring plasma salicylate levels and acid-base balance is critical to guide further treatment decisions.

For local anesthetic toxicity, lipid emulsion therapy has proven effective, particularly in cases involving lidocaine or bupivacaine. This therapy works by creating a "lipid sink," binding lipophilic drugs to reduce active drug levels. The recommended protocol begins with a bolus dose of 1.5 mL/kg over one minute, followed by a maintenance infusion of 15 mL/kg/hour. The maximum cumulative dose should not exceed 12 mL/kg. However, this therapy remains unlicensed for overdose treatment, and safety concerns regarding rapid infusion persist.

In calcium channel blocker or beta-blocker poisoning, insulin therapy is employed to counteract drug-induced hypotension. Treatment involves administering 1 unit/kg of short-acting insulin intravenously, followed by a maintenance infusion of 0.5–2 units/kg/hour. This approach supports hemodynamic stability.

For cases of severe poisoning, such as methanol, ethylene glycol, or lithium toxicity, advanced techniques like hemodialysis may be necessary to enhance toxin elimination. Hemodialysis is also beneficial in salicylate and phenobarbital poisoning. Although rarely required, hemoperfusion may assist in cases involving severe barbiturate or chloral hydrate toxicity.

Healthcare providers should remain vigilant for delayed effects of poisons and antidotes, ensuring continuous monitoring and accurate documentation of therapies. Consultation with specialists is strongly recommended for rare or complex cases to optimize patient outcomes and adhere to evidence-based practices.

Plasma Paracetamol (mg/L).   Plasma Paracetamol (mmol/L)

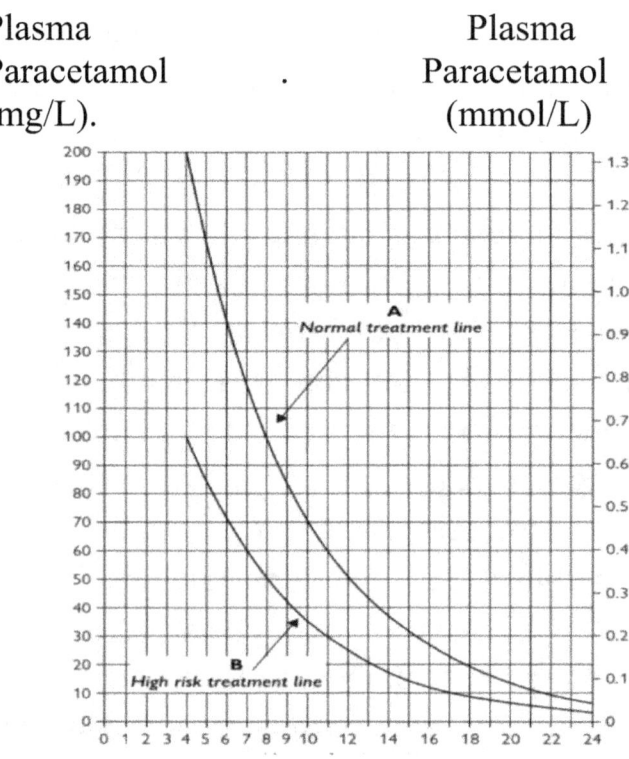

House after ingestion

Figure 4-1: Paracetamol treatment graph

Paracetamol Overdose Management

Line A: Standard treatment for most patients.

Line B: For high-risk groups, including those with malnutrition, chronic alcoholism, HIV, cystic fibrosis, or taking anticonvulsants, rifampicin, or St. John's wort.

Note: Confirm if lab results use mg/L or mmol/L. Start treatment immediately if overdose timing is unclear or plasma levels are near the treatment threshold.

Management of Tricyclic Antidepressant Overdose

Causes and Symptoms
Anticholinergic toxicity commonly arises from tricyclic antidepressant overdose but may also result from substances like procyclidine or atropine (e.g., in Atropa belladonna).

Key symptoms include:

Tachycardia, dry mouth, dry skin, dilated pupils, urinary retention, ataxia, and jerky limb movements.

Severe cases can lead to coma, muscle tone abnormalities, respiratory depression, and convulsions.

Post-coma, patients may experience delirium, hallucinations, severe dysarthria, and jerky limb movements.

ECG Changes

Sinus tachycardia is common; prolonged PR interval and QRS duration indicate severe poisoning.

Rhythm may mimic ventricular tachycardia (VT) but often represents sinus tachycardia with conduction delay.

Severe cases may involve ventricular arrhythmias, bradycardia, and potentially fatal cardio-respiratory depression.

Treatment Protocol

1. Supportive Care

Secure the airway, intubate, and provide ventilation as needed.

Continuous monitoring due to the risk of rapid deterioration.

2. Activated Charcoal

Administer if more than 4 mg/kg was ingested within one hour, provided the airway is secure.

3. Convulsions

Single, brief seizures usually do not require treatment.

For prolonged or frequent seizures, use IV lorazepam or diazepam.

4. Arrhythmias

Address hypoxia and acidosis.

Sodium bicarbonate (8.4%) IV (adult: 50–100 mL; child: 1 mL/kg) can improve cardiac function and reduce toxicity. Aim for arterial pH 7.5–7.55, avoiding pH >7.65.

Consult specialists if arrhythmias persist despite treatment.

5. Hypotension

Elevate the patient's legs and provide IV fluids.

Glucagon or dopamine (2–10 mcg/kg/min) may be necessary in refractory cases under specialist guidance.

6. Additional Measures

Lipid emulsion therapy (Intralipid®) may be considered for severe cardiac toxicity.

Avoid using physostigmine or flumazenil due to seizure risks.

Recovery

Most patients regain consciousness within 36 hours, though delirium and hallucinations can persist for several days, requiring oral diazepam for sedation.

ECG Changes in Tricyclic Antidepressant Poisoning

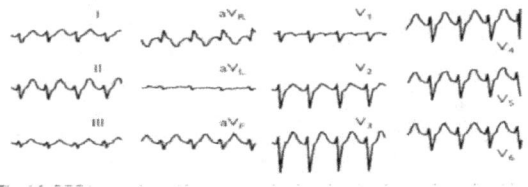

Figure 4-2: ECG in Tricyclic Antidepressant Poisoning

Displays sinus tachycardia with prolonged conduction intervals, often misinterpreted as ventricular tachycardia (VT).

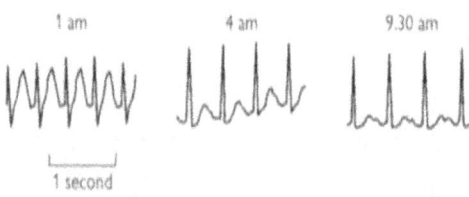

Figure 4-3: Serial ECG in Amitriptyline Poisoning

Rhythm strips demonstrating spontaneous recovery with supportive management.

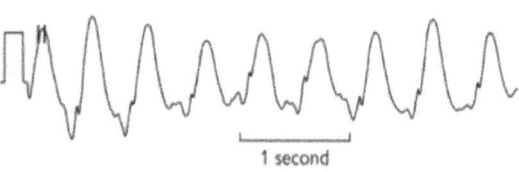

Figure 4-4: Severe Tricyclic Antidepressant Poisoning: ECG Findings

ECG from a critically poisoned patient with GCS 3, requiring intubation and ventilation, and presenting with hypotension (BP 70/50 mmHg).

Benzodiazepine Toxicity

Overview: Benzodiazepines (e.g., diazepam, nitrazepam, temazepam) are rarely life-threatening when overdosed alone but significantly enhance the effects of other central nervous system (CNS) depressants like alcohol, tricyclic antidepressants, or barbiturates.

Clinical Presentation:

Common symptoms: Drowsiness, dizziness, ataxia, dysarthria.

Severe cases: Coma, respiratory depression, mild hypotension (more likely in elderly individuals or those with chronic COPD).

Fatal outcomes are rare and typically associated with respiratory failure.

Management:

1. Initial Steps:

Ensure a patent airway and assist ventilation if necessary.

Administer activated charcoal within 1 hour of a toxic dose.

2. Supportive Care:

Monitor for prolonged motor and cognitive impairment due to long-acting metabolites.

Warn patients about potential delays in resuming activities such as driving.

3. Specific Antidote:

Flumazenil: Effective within 1 minute but short-acting (<1 hour). Use with caution due to risks of seizures, cardiac arrhythmias, or withdrawal in benzodiazepine-dependent patients. Avoid mixed benzodiazepine and tricyclic poisoning, as it may precipitate convulsions or cardiac arrest.

Clomethiazole Toxicity

Clinical Features:

Common signs: Coma, respiratory depression, muscle tone

Theophylline Poisoning

Theophylline and aminophylline are medications that can lead to fatal poisoning, particularly when slow-release formulations are ingested. Toxicity may not manifest until 12 to 24 hours post-ingestion, requiring careful observation during this period.

Clinical Features

Patients typically present with nausea, severe vomiting (which often does not respond to antiemetics), abdominal pain, and in some cases, haematemesis. Other symptoms include restlessness, muscle hypertonia, hyperreflexia, headaches, and convulsions. Severe poisoning can lead to coma, hyperventilation, hyperpyrexia, rhabdomyolysis, and arrhythmias (starting with sinus tachycardia, possibly progressing to supraventricular or ventricular arrhythmias, and even ventricular fibrillation). Blood pressure may be elevated initially but can decrease in severe cases. Metabolic disturbances include respiratory alkalosis, followed by metabolic acidosis, hyperglycaemia, hypokalaemia, and hypomagnesaemia.

Management

Supportive care: Close monitoring of ECG, heart rate, and blood pressure.

Laboratory investigations: Measure electrolytes (U&E), calcium, magnesium, phosphate, glucose, ABG, and plasma theophylline levels. Repeated measurements of potassium are essential for correcting hypokalemia, as this can help prevent arrhythmias. Potassium should be corrected at no faster than 20 mmol/hr.

Gastric decontamination: Consider gastric lavage if less than 1 hour since ingestion. Activated charcoal may also be given, preferably via an NG tube if vomiting is severe.

Antiemetic treatment: Ondansetron (8 mg slow IV in adults) can help control intractable vomiting.

Manage GI bleeding: Blood transfusions and ranitidine may be required for GI bleeding.

Cardiac management: For tachycardia with adequate cardiac output, avoid treatment. Non-selective beta-blockers (e.g., propranolol) may help with arrhythmias, but caution is necessary in asthmatic patients. Lidocaine and mexiletine should be avoided, as they may precipitate seizures. Disopyramide is the preferred antiarrhythmic for ventricular arrhythmias.

Seizure control: Administer diazepam or lorazepam for convulsions.

Advanced therapies: For severe poisoning, consider charcoal hemoperfusion or haemodialysis, particularly if activated charcoal administration is difficult due to vomiting.

Monitor potassium levels closely during recovery as large amounts of potassium administered initially can lead to hyperkalemia.

Salbutamol Poisoning

Overdose with β2-agonists, such as salbutamol, may lead to symptoms including vomiting, agitation, tremor, tachycardia, palpitations, hypokalaemia, and hypertension. Rarely, severe complications like hallucinations, hyperglycaemia, delayed hypoglycemia, ventricular arrhythmias, myocardial ischaemia, and convulsions can occur.

Management

Supportive care: Correct hypokalemia with intravenous potassium (maximum infusion rate of 20 mmol/hr).

Monitor vital signs: ECG and blood pressure should be closely monitored.

Decontamination: Activated charcoal may reduce drug absorption if administered soon after ingestion.

Cardiac management: Tachycardia should not be treated if there is an adequate cardiac output. If severe tachyarrhythmias or hypokalaemia develop, beta-blockers like metoprolol or esmolol may be used but must be avoided in asthmatic patients to prevent bronchospasm.

Iron Poisoning

Iron poisoning is often seen in children, as iron tablets may resemble candy. While fatalities are uncommon, severe poisoning can occur, especially with slow-release formulations, which contain between 35–105 mg of elemental iron per tablet.

Clinical Features

In the initial hours, common symptoms include nausea, vomiting, diarrhea, and abdominal pain. Vomit and stools may appear gray or black and could contain blood. Hyperglycemia and elevated white blood cell count (WCC) may occur. In severe cases, haematemesis, drowsiness, convulsions, and coma may develop. After 6-12 hours, early symptoms may subside, but a worsening phase can occur between 24-48 hours, presenting with shock, hypoglycaemia, jaundice, metabolic acidosis, hepatic encephalopathy, renal failure, and potentially bowel infarction. Survivors may experience long-term complications such as gastric strictures or pyloric obstruction.

Management

Supportive care: Monitor serum iron levels, FBC, glucose, liver function tests (LFTs), INR, and ABGs.

Gastric decontamination: Activated charcoal is ineffective in iron poisoning. Whole-bowel irrigation may be indicated, especially if slow-release iron preparations are ingested.

Expert advice: In cases of severe poisoning, deferoxamine, an iron chelator, should be administered intravenously (15 mg/kg/hr up to 80 mg/kg total). This treatment is essential even before serum iron concentrations are available.

Desferrioxamine side effects: Rapid infusion can cause hypotension, while prolonged use may lead to rashes, anaphylaxis, pulmonary oedema, or ARDS.

Urine monitoring: The iron-desferrioxamine complex will color the urine orange or red, which confirms that the iron has been bound.

Discharge criteria: If no symptoms appear within 6 hours, patients may be discharged, but should return if new symptoms develop.

Pregnancy: Pregnancy does not alter the need for desferrioxamine in cases of severe poisoning.

Ethanol Poisoning

Ethanol ingestion may initially cause disinhibition, followed by ataxia, dizziness, dysarthria, and drowsiness. It potentiates the effects of other CNS depressants. Severe intoxication may result in coma, respiratory depression, hypotension, hypothermia, and metabolic acidosis, with hypoglycemia being a particular concern in children. Fatality may result from respiratory failure or aspiration.

Management

Airway management: Ensure the airway is clear and the patient is positioned to prevent aspiration.

Blood glucose monitoring: Check glucose every 1-2 hours. Correct hypoglycemia with glucose (do not use glucagon unless IV access is unavailable).

Head injury evaluation: Be vigilant for signs of trauma, particularly head injuries. A CT brain scan may be warranted for patients who are comatose or have focal neurological signs.

Poison co-ingestion: Other ingested substances should be treated accordingly.

Gastric decontamination: Activated charcoal and gastric lavage are ineffective for ethanol intoxication.

ICU care: Severe cases may require ICU admission for supportive care and potentially dialysis.

Methanol Poisoning

Methanol toxicity arises from the metabolites formaldehyde and formic acid. Even small ingestions can result in blindness (10mL) or death (30mL).

Clinical Features

Initial symptoms include mild drowsiness, followed by more serious symptoms 12-24 hours later: vomiting, abdominal pain, headache, dizziness, blurred vision, and progression to coma. Metabolic acidosis, hyperglycaemia, and elevated serum amylase are common. Long-term effects include permanent blindness and Parkinsonism.

Management

Gastric decontamination: If ingestion occurred within the past hour, consider gastric lavage, but do not administer charcoal.

Laboratory investigations: Measure ABG, U&E, glucose, LFTs, ethanol, and plasma methanol levels, if available. Calculate the osmolar gap and anion gap.

Toxicology consultation: Contact a poisons information center for expert advice.

Fomepizole or ethanol: Early administration of fomepizole or ethanol can mitigate methanol toxicity, especially in patients with metabolic acidosis and a high anion gap.

Sodium bicarbonate: Use to correct metabolic acidosis, aiming for a pH of 7.44. Caution against hypernatraemia if large doses are needed.

acid: Administer 30 mg IV every 6 hours for 48 hours.

Dialysis: Consider ICU referral for severe poisoning and possible haemodialysis.

Ethylene Glycol Poisoning

Overview
Ethylene glycol is primarily used as an antifreeze and is highly toxic when ingested. The fatal dose for an adult is approximately 100g, or 90mL of pure ethylene glycol. The toxic effects are caused by its metabolites, including glycolaldehyde, glycolic acid, and oxalic acid. Treatment options such as fomepizole or ethanol can inhibit the metabolism of ethylene glycol, preventing its toxic effects.

Clinical Features

Initial Phase (0-12 hours): Symptoms resemble drunkenness, without the typical smell of alcohol. Common signs include ataxia, dysarthria, nausea, vomiting, and sometimes hematemesis. Seizures, coma, and severe metabolic acidosis can follow.

Secondary Phase (12-24 hours): Hyperventilation, pulmonary edema, tachycardia, arrhythmias, and cardiac failure can occur. Hypocalcemia can become severe.

Renal Phase (24-72 hours): Acute tubular necrosis and renal failure are observed, often accompanied by cranial nerve palsies.

Diagnostic Finding: Calcium oxalate monohydrate crystals in the urine are indicative of ethylene glycol poisoning. Additionally, some antifreeze brands contain fluorescein, which causes urine to fluoresce under UV light, assisting in diagnosis.

Management

1. Initial Steps:

Gastric Lavage: Consider if the patient ingested within the last hour, but avoid activated charcoal.

Laboratory Tests: Measure arterial blood gasses (ABG), electrolytes, glucose, liver function, and osmolality. Calculate the osmolar gap and anion gap.

Monitoring: Observe the patient for at least 6 hours, even if asymptomatic, and monitor ECG, blood pressure, pulse, and urine output.

2. Medical Intervention:

Fomepizole or Ethanol: Administer as early as possible to block metabolism of ethylene glycol.

If fomepizole is unavailable, administer ethanol (2.5 mL/kg orally or 10 mL/kg intravenously).

Sodium Bicarbonate: Correct metabolic acidosis if ventilation and fluid resuscitation are inadequate.

Calcium Gluconate: Administer if hypocalcemia is severe, especially with seizures or prolonged QT intervals, though it should be used cautiously due to the risk of calcium oxalate stone formation.

Hemodialysis: Consider severe poisoning, particularly if there is high blood ethylene glycol concentration.

Paraquat Poisoning

Overview
Paraquat is a potent herbicide, and ingestion of just 10mL can lead to fatal outcomes. Although rare in the UK due to regulatory restrictions,

paraquat poisoning remains a concern in other regions.

Clinical Features

Immediate Symptoms: Upon ingestion, paraquat causes burning pain in the mouth and throat, nausea, vomiting, and abdominal pain.

Progression (within 24 hours): Large ingestions lead to rapid deterioration, including shock, pulmonary edema, and metabolic acidosis, followed by coma and convulsions.

Pulmonary Damage: Pulmonary fibrosis develops 5–7 days post-ingestion, manifesting as breathlessness, cyanosis, and lung shadowing visible on chest X-ray. Hypoxic death may occur 7–14 days post-exposure.

Management

Avoid Oxygen Supplementation: This can worsen pulmonary toxicity.

Activated Charcoal: Consider if within 1 hour of ingestion.

Gastric Lavage: Avoid, as it may cause esophageal perforation.

Prognosis Testing: Measure lactate levels as they are indicative of prognosis, and send urine samples for paraquat testing.

Monitor: Continuous monitoring for signs of lung damage and other complications.

Petrol and Paraffin Poisoning

Overview
Petrol, paraffin (kerosene), and similar hydrocarbons can lead to poisoning if ingested or aspirated, with pneumonitis being the major

complication. This is often seen when fuels are stored improperly or siphoned from vehicles.

Clinical Features

Initial Symptoms: May be asymptomatic, or there may be nausea, vomiting, and diarrhea.

Aspiration Symptoms: Coughing, wheezing, breathlessness, and cyanosis are common, along with fever. Chest X-ray may reveal pneumonitis.

Severe Symptoms: Pulmonary edema, drowsiness, convulsions, or coma may develop in severe cases.

Management

Gastric Lavage: Avoid, as it can worsen aspiration risk.

Chest X-ray: Obtain after 6-8 hours, sooner if necessary.

Supportive Care: Provide oxygen, bronchodilators, and steroids as needed. Consider CPAP/IPPV for patients showing respiratory failure.

Organophosphate Poisoning

Overview
Organophosphates, widely used as insecticides, inhibit cholinesterase activity, leading to excessive acetylcholine accumulation at nerve endings. Symptoms and severity vary depending on the compound and exposure.

Clinical Features

Mild Exposure: Symptoms may include anxiety, nausea, sweating, miosis, and abdominal discomfort.

Severe Exposure: Respiratory failure, bronchospasm, convulsions, and coma can occur, with delayed symptoms appearing 1-4 days after exposure.

Chronic Effects: Muscle weakness, cranial nerve palsies, and peripheral neuropathy may develop.

Management

1. Personal Protection: Ensure all involved in patient care wear protective clothing.

2. Supportive Treatment: Maintain the airway, give oxygen, and manage convulsions with diazepam.

3. Atropine: Administer for bronchospasm and secretions. The dose may need to be titrated based on symptoms.

4. Pralidoxime: Use for moderate to severe poisoning. Start with an IV bolus, followed by continuous infusion.

5. NPIS Consultation: Discuss antidote availability and treatment protocols with the National Poisons Information Service.

Cyanide Poisoning

Overview

Cyanide is a potent toxin that inhibits cellular respiration, often causing death within minutes upon inhalation. Cyanide compounds may also be ingested or absorbed through the skin.

Clinical Features

Early Symptoms: Dizziness, headache, palpitations, breathlessness, and drowsiness.

Severe Poisoning: Coma, convulsions, cyanosis (rare), pulmonary edema, arrhythmias, and cardiorespiratory failure.

Classic Sign: A bitter almond odor on the breath, though not everyone can detect it.

Management

1. Initial Steps: Remove contaminated clothing and wash exposed skin.

2. Oxygen Therapy: Administer 100% oxygen to manage hypoxia.

3. Activated Charcoal/Gastric Lavage: Consider if ingestion occurred within 1 hour.

4. Specific Antidotes: Use sodium thiosulfate or sodium nitrite for mild to moderate poisoning. In severe cases, dicobalt edetate may be administered, though this carries risks.

5. Symptom Monitoring: Constant ECG monitoring and supportive care are essential.

Chemical incidents, which may involve one or more casualties, can stem from accidental releases (e.g., chlorine gas) or deliberate acts (e.g., terrorist attacks). These events share common features with other types of CBRN (chemical, biological, radiological, and nuclear) incidents. The management of such incidents requires rapid, organized action. Here's a step-by-step guide for healthcare providers:

1. Notify senior ED staff immediately if a chemical incident is suspected.

2. Avoid contamination of other patients and staff.

3. Wear appropriate personal protective equipment (PPE) unless the patient has been decontaminated prior.

4. Decontaminate the patient following established protocols if this has not already been done (see page 218 for more details on patient decontamination).

5. Perform resuscitation as needed, addressing the airway, breathing, and circulation.

6. Assess clinical symptoms and identify the toxic agent involved.

7. Administer antidotes as appropriate and reassess the patient's condition.

8. Confirm if additional casualties are expected and inform the relevant teams.

9. Notify the local health protection team and seek advice from experts via TOXBASE (National Poisons Information Service) or the Department for Environment, Food, and Rural Affairs (Defra) for CBRN emergency situations.

10. If there is suspicion of a deliberate release, inform the police and engage relevant agencies, including public relations personnel.

Common chemicals involved in such incidents include chlorine, cyanide, organophosphates, and CS gas (tear gas), all of which have specific toxic effects and antidotes (see the respective sections in the manual for detailed management).

In the case of chemical incidents, collaboration with NPIS and reference to TOXBASE can provide crucial information regarding the toxicity of various chemicals and the appropriate treatment options. Key details are provided about 60 chemicals that may be deliberately released, including guidance on managing the associated risks and symptoms.

Decontamination of Patients

After exposure to a hazardous substance, the goal of decontamination is to minimize the risks to both the patient and others. In many cases, initial decontamination occurs at the scene, but patients may arrive at the emergency department (ED) without warning, requiring immediate action. It is crucial to address contamination fears, as some individuals may not be at actual risk. Organizing the ED effectively, ensuring 'clean' areas remain uncontaminated, and maintaining communication between the decontamination team and the ED staff are vital in these high-pressure scenarios.

Toxicity from Plants, Berries, and Mushrooms

Plant and Berry Toxicity

Although many children are inclined to eat plant leaves or colorful berries, serious poisoning from plants is rare. When identifying plants, use reference books and seek advice from Poison Information Services. Most garden and house plants are non-toxic and do not require intervention after ingestion. A rare example is poisoning from laburnum, which may cause mild symptoms such as nausea and vomiting. However, serious poisoning is exceedingly rare, and no specific treatment is needed unless severe symptoms occur.

Mushroom Poisoning

While most mushroom-related poisonings are not fatal, the ingestion of the Amanita (death cap mushroom) can be life-threatening. The primary symptoms of mushroom poisoning typically appear within 6-12 hours after ingestion. The diagnosis hinges on the timing of symptom onset, with Amanita poisoning leading to vomiting, diarrhea, liver, and renal failure after a latent period. Management focuses on symptomatic care, and activated charcoal may be used within 1 hour of ingestion to reduce absorption. In cases of suspected Amanita poisoning, immediate expert advice should be sought.

Button Battery Ingestion

Children frequently swallow button or disc batteries, which can get lodged in the esophagus, leading to perforation or stenosis. If the battery reaches the stomach, it typically passes through the digestive system without issues. However, batteries in the esophagus require immediate endoscopic removal to prevent severe injury. X-rays or metal detectors can confirm the presence and location of swallowed batteries. If the battery is stuck in the stomach for more than two days, referral for endoscopic removal may be necessary. Most batteries that pass into the intestines will naturally pass within 1-2 weeks, although close monitoring is needed for any signs of complications such as abdominal pain or bleeding.

Ingestion of Magnets
When children ingest magnets, especially multiple magnets or when combined with a ferro metallic object, it can cause bowel necrosis or perforation. Immediate removal of the magnets is required to prevent life-threatening complications.

Novel Psychoactive Substances (NPS)
NPS, once referred to as "legal highs," include a range of substances that mimic the effects of illegal drugs such as cocaine, cannabis, or ecstasy. These substances are often combined with alcohol or other drugs, which can exacerbate their effects. The four main types of NPS are stimulants, synthetic cannabinoids, depressants, and hallucinogens.

1. Stimulant NPS (e.g., mephedrone) can cause symptoms similar to amphetamines, such as agitation, tachycardia, and hypertension. Treatment is similar to that for MDMA/amphetamine toxicity.

2. Cannabinoid NPS (e.g., "spice") can lead to agitation or confusion, and symptoms may resemble those of cannabis intoxication. Symptomatic management is often required.

3. Depressant NPS can result in reduced consciousness, hypoventilation, and bradycardia, necessitating treatment similar to benzodiazepine or opioid poisoning.

4. Hallucinogenic NPS may cause psychedelic effects, which require treatment similar to LSD or ketamine toxicity.

For all cases of NPS exposure, supportive care is crucial, and identifying the specific toxidrome helps guide treatment. Patients who are asymptomatic after four hours and have not required treatment are generally considered safe to discharge.

Recreational Drug Toxicity

Toxicity from recreational drugs such as heroin, cocaine, and ecstasy can vary in severity. These drugs may be mixed with other substances, leading to unpredictable effects. It's essential to be aware of the varied presentation of illicit drug toxicity, which may involve symptoms like agitation, hyperthermia, or seizures. Addressing the specific toxidrome and providing appropriate symptomatic care are critical for managing these emergencies.

References

1. Tintinalli's Emergency Medicine: A Comprehensive Study Guide
Tintinalli JE, Stapczynski J, Ma OJ, Yealy DM, Meckler GD.
Latest Edition. McGraw Hill Education.
A foundational text covering the full spectrum of emergency medical care.

2. Rosen's Emergency Medicine: Concepts and Clinical Practice
Walls RM, Hockberger RS, Gausche-Hill M.
Latest Edition. Elsevier.
A comprehensive resource offering in-depth discussions on emergency medicine principles and advanced case management.

3. The Advanced Trauma Life Support (ATLS) Manual
American College of Surgeons.
Current Edition.

A step-by-step guide for managing trauma patients, including primary and secondary assessments.

4. Emergency Medicine Procedures
Reichman EF.
Latest Edition. McGraw Hill.
A detailed procedural guide for emergency interventions.

5. Handbook of Critical and Intensive Care Medicine
Marino PL.
Current Edition. Springer.
Focuses on the critical care aspects often encountered in emergency medicine settings.

6. Poisoning and Drug Overdose
Olson KR.
Latest Edition. McGraw Hill.
A concise guide on managing toxicology and poisoning cases in emergency settings.

7. Emergency Medicine Manual

Ma OJ, Mateer JR.
Latest Edition. McGraw Hill.
A quick-reference manual for emergency department protocols and best practices.

8. Clinical Emergency Medicine Casebook
Eisenberg RL, Bell J.
Latest Edition. Cambridge University Press.
A case-based approach to learning and applying emergency medicine principles.

9. Practical Emergency Resuscitation and Critical Care
Shiber JR, Green RS.
Latest Edition. Cambridge University Press.
Provides practical approaches to resuscitation and critical care management.

10. Textbook of Adult Emergency Medicine
Cameron P, Jelinek GA, Kelly A-M, et al.
Latest Edition. Elsevier.
A comprehensive guide to emergency medical practices, tailored to adult care.

11. The 5-Minute Emergency Medicine Consult
Schaider JJ, Hayden SR, Wolfe RE, Barkin RM.
Latest Edition. Wolters Kluwer.
A concise and quick-reference guide for emergency medicine practitioners.

12. Evidence-Based Emergency Care: Diagnostic Testing and Clinical Decision Rules
Carpenter CR, Raja AS, et al.
Latest Edition. Wiley-Blackwell.
Focused on evidence-based practices and diagnostic testing in emergency settings.

13. Advanced Cardiovascular Life Support (ACLS) Provider Manual
American Heart Association.
Current Edition.
Authoritative guidelines for managing cardiac emergencies and advanced life support.

www.ingramcontent.com/pod-product-compliance
Lightning Source LLC
Chambersburg PA
CBHW071017240526
45469CB00006BD/1950